Sexual
Sorcery

Sexual Sorcery

A COMPLETE GUIDE TO SEX MAGICK

Jason Augustus Newcomb

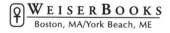
WEISER BOOKS
Boston, MA/York Beach, ME

First published in 2005 by
Red Wheel/Weiser, LLC
York Beach, ME
With offices at:
368 Congress Street
Boston, MA 02210
www.redwheelweiser.com

Library of Congress Cataloging-in-Publication Data

Newcomb, Jason Augustus.
    Sexual sorcery : a complete guide to sex magick / Jason Augustus
Newcomb.
        p. cm.
    Includes bibliographical references.
    ISBN 1-57863-330-3
        1. Magic. 2. Sex—Miscellanea. I. Title.
    BF1623.S4N49 2005
    133.4'3—dc22   2005008893

Typeset in Bembo, ITC Legacy Sans, DIN Neuzeit Grotesk and
Bodega Sans.

Printed in the Canada
TCP

12 11 10 09 08 07 06 05
  8 7 6 5 4 3 2 1

TO JENNIFER,
MY HEART AND MY INSPIRATION

CONTENTS

ACKNOWLEDGMENTS

I want to sincerely thank the ton of people who have helped in the creation of this manual, but I'm only able to mention a few in this place.

Thanks especially to my mom, even though I'm sure she'll hate this book.

Many thanks to Mike Conlon for being a wonderful editor and supporter of my work. And a thousand thanks to all of the excellent folks at Red Wheel/Weiser.

Thanks to Patrick for selling me a copy of Louis Culling's *A Manual of Sex Magick* many years ago. Thanks to Barbara for letting me pay too much for it, so that I could avoid "haggling over the price of an egg from a perfectly black hen."

Thanks to Lon Duquette for telling me that writing about sex magick was not a mortal sin, and to Fratres Hymeneaus Beta and Sabazius for (hopefully) not throwing me out of the O.T.O.

Thanks to Jennifer for your tireless support and love in my field research.

Thanks to all of the women who suffered in my early learning curve, and to all of the women who answered my highly invasive questions about female sexuality.

Thanks to River for her ears and eyes.

Thanks to Scott Lesser, because nearly all great books acknowledge him.

And most especially, thanks to Robert J. Maiolo for returning my coat.

The Tau and the circle together make one form of the Rosy Cross, the uniting of subject and object which is the Great Work, and which is symbolized sometimes as this cross and circle, sometimes as the Lingam-Yoni, sometimes as the Ankh or Crux Ansata, sometimes by the Spire and Nave of a church or temple, and sometimes as a marriage feast, mystic marriage, spiritual marriage, "chymical nuptials," and in a hundred other ways. Whatever the form chosen, it is the symbol of the Great Work.

—*Aleister Crowley*

Once they are coupled together, and if this crime of prostitution were not bad enough for them, they offer their infamy to the heavens: the man and the woman gather the man's sperm in their hands, raise their eyes to heaven, and with their hands full of their uncleanness, offer it to the father saying: "We offer you this gift, the body of Christ." Then they eat of it and take communion with their own sperm, saying: "Here is the body of Christ, here is the Paschal Lamb for which they confess the passion of Christ." They do the same with the women's menstruation. They collect the blood of her impurity and take communion with it in the same manner.

—*St. Epiphanius of Salamis*

If a man ardently wishes a force or power into being and guards this wish from the instant that he penetrates into the woman until the instant that he withdraws from her, his wish is necessarily fulfilled.

—*Paschal Beverly Randolph*

Thou hast ravished my heart, my sister, my spouse; thou hast ravished my heart with one of thine eyes, with one chain of thy neck.
How fair is thy love, my sister, my spouse! how much better is thy love than wine! and the smell of thine ointments than all spices!
Thy lips, O my spouse, drop as the honeycomb: honey and milk are under thy tongue; and the smell of thy garments is like the smell of Lebanon.

—*Song of Solomon, 4, 9-11*

INTRODUCTION

I love you! I yearn to you! Pale or purple, veiled or voluptuous, I who am all pleasure and purple, and drunkenness of the inner-most sense, desire you. Put on the wings, and arouse the coiled splendour within you: come unto me!

—*Liber AL vel Legis, I, 61*

So, you'd like to be a sexual sorcerer? Perhaps you want to learn the true secrets of sex magick, or magnetically draw sexual partners to yourself, or become more accomplished in bed, or improve your orgasms, or even achieve spiritual transcendence through sex. You can learn all of that and more in this book. But this is, first and foremost, a book about love. It is a valentine to the divine lover, and to all of the earthly women I have adored. Because its theme is love, this book may seem a touch more lyrical and mystical in places than my previous works. But this is a practical book of sex magick. It will lead you systematically and directly to heights of sexual power, ecstasy, and illumination.

This is not a book of philosophy, though I will discuss some of the philosophy behind sex magick. My main interest here is to provide you with a practical gateway into exploring the powerful energies of sexual magick through love. This is not a dry history book, though I will briefly discuss some of the long and winding history of sexual magick throughout the world. Nor is this book an anachronistic fantasy. I will not attempt to rebuild the sexual temples of Mesopotamia, the secret libertine lodges of medieval times, or even the hedonistic sacred rites of Tantra. This is a book for the sexual magician of the twenty-first century. Our own cultural landscape is the ground we must sexually sanctify and imbue with sexual power. And it is love itself that will sanctify our work.

There is no limit to love. There is no incorrect love. Love suffers no rules or restrictions. It is free to travel through all the planes—the highest and the lowest—and to every darkened corner of the Earth and the cosmos. In the words of St. Paul: "Love is patient, love is kind. It is not jealous, is not inflated, it is not rude, it does not seek its own interests, it is not quick-tempered. It does not rejoice over wrongdoing but rejoices with the truth. It bears all things, believes all things, hopes all things, endures all things" (I Corinthians 13: 4-7). True love is simply divine love. Divine love is simply true love—love given without expectation. Love alone is eternal, creating and destroying each unit of itself in a never-ending dance of ecstasy.

Love is the universal formula of both creation and spiritual illumination, the return to our own divine source. Each unit of creation is the coition of two individual forces, resulting in a new third force that contains both the originals in a new way. For instance, I feel like creating a painting, but have no ideas about what to paint. Suddenly, inspiration strikes and I know what I will paint. This is the coition. The resulting painting will be a new individual, containing elements of both the unconscious inspiration that set me to work and elements of my conscious individuality. This same dynamic drives chemistry, mathematics, religion, and magick. He who has ears, let him hear.

All is love. Aleister Crowley once wrote, "the formula is now love in all cases. . ."[1] The second knowledge lecture of the Hermetic Order of the Golden Dawn points this out very succinctly and beautifully in its observation that the glyph of Venus is the only symbol that encompasses the whole Tree of Life—from Kether, the crown, the divine monad, to Malkuth, the kingdom of the material world.

Venus is a sexual goddess, and sexuality is inherent in love, as it is in all things. In my last book, I described the universe as a great mind,[2] and this is indeed one way of looking at the divine. However, the divine can also be described as a great phallus (for instance, the *Shiva-lingam*) or, more accurately, as a great phallus and a great *kteis* conjoined, ever locked in the act of creation.

Likewise, the sexual aspect of the spiritual world is revealed simply in the facts of nature. New life is the result of sex. In fact, the worship of generative power seems to be at the root of the earliest religions, those that are the simplest and, perhaps, the most accurate. Even when cultures did not fully understand the connection between the sexual act

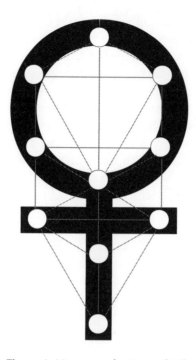

Figure 1. Venus on the Tree of Life

and procreation, both of these processes were viewed as inherently sacred. Sexual energy is the energy of the universe. It is the energy of desire, creativity, magnetism, gravity, starlight—the energy of existence itself. Love is at the core of all these.

All religions and all magical acts are inherently sexual, because the universe is sexual. Polarity exists from the beginning in the *yin* and the *yang*, the *Logos* and the *Sophia*, Shakti and Shiva, Nuit and Hadit, Babalon and the Seven-Headed Beast whereon she rides. Religious experiences are universally ecstatic, the merging of any or all of these polarities into unity, into an explosive consciousness of their essential oneness. Perception is the relation of self and not-self, and the union of these is a sexual union. The point of perception intersects with the infinite circle of perceivable experiences and information, and each union is an ecstatic coition of consciousness.

The sex drive itself contains a yearning for transcendence. No moment is more powerfully and immediately ecstatic in the life of the average human being than the moment of physical orgasm. This moment contains an immense amount of physical power; unmistakably, unambiguously, this is a moment of incredible force and wonder. How much more true will this be for a person who has transformed that orgasm into a true union with the power of the divine?

Sex has an extremely powerful effect on consciousness, so sex magick is extremely powerful. Sexuality can be confusing, emotionally unsafe, and painful. The same can be said of sex magick. Whatever issues you have about sex will quickly come up as soon as you begin exploring sex magick. Sex magick is often considered the most powerful method of manifesting physical results in your magick. In this book, you will fully explore these practical uses of magick, as well as the more mystical uses for sexuality. You can learn many things here: how to be a better lover, how to attract lovers, how to improve your sex drive and sexual vigor, how to achieve "gnosis" through sex, and how to accomplish magical miracles with your enhanced sexual power.

This book speaks very frankly and explicitly about a wide range of sexual activities, and I reveal in its pages many of my own sexual peccadilloes and perhaps bizarre-sounding ideas. If you have issues around sex or think it is somehow immoral or strange to combine sexuality with spirituality and magical practices, this is definitely not a book you will enjoy. Since the title of this book is very unambiguous, I doubt that anything in it will take you by surprise. You may, however, come up against hidden taboos and restrictions in your personality, deeply indwelling uncharted regions of your psyche, and you may need to examine yourself thoroughly.

Sacred Sexual Energy

The use of sexual energy for sacred purposes was long a guarded secret within almost all of the world's religious and magical movements. It has been known for ages that to cast the pearls of sexual gnosis before swine—the repressed, imbalanced, and dysfunctional masses that comprise the majority of humanity—is to court disaster. At best, sexual magick is viewed by the masses as a derangement or a perversion; at worst it is partially understood, and used for selfish and ultimately destructive ends such as psychic vampirism, manipulation, or enslavement to lower desires. Sexual energy is so powerful that it can swiftly bring you to the highest spiritual heights and give you the greatest gifts of insight and power. Used improperly, it can tear your very soul from your body and turn you into the weakest slave of the crudest and lowliest astral larvae in the gloomiest corners of Hades. I have personally experienced both.

Early Christians, Tantric yogis, pagan mystery schools, Taoists, Buddhists, ancient Egyptian priestly classes, Hebrew Kabbalists—all these traditions contained sexual teachings. These sexual practices did not form the basis of the whole religion, however; rather, they were reserved for a chosen few. There were sometimes two different traditions—one libertine and one ascetic—within the same broad religious culture. Most of the faithful were taught that the highest illumination and spiritual insight was attainable only through renunciation of all bodily pleasures and desires, and complete mental, moral, and physical continence. But the elect were informed that the fastest, and perhaps best, way to achieve this same gnosis was through a careful cultivation of these very desires, and a conscious directing of this sexual power toward ecstatic spiritual heights.

Chastity and promiscuity are both inherently grounded in sexual energy—the former passively and inwardly, the latter actively and outwardly. Both can lead to illumination, and both can easily lead to delusion and ugliness. When chastity and moral taboos are encouraged as the ideal, however, society is much more easily controlled. They are, therefore, often used as tools by those in authority. After all, if everyone explored the farthest reaches of their consciousness through all sorts of outlandish practices, tearing away limitations, repression, and binding social conditioning from their minds and hearts, the social structure of the community would become quite unstable. Actively sexual teachings were kept secret, confined to inner sanctuaries where advanced souls used them for real religious evolution. The outward teachings of chastity and repression served largely to control the out-of-balance sexual impulses of the masses. Many sexual sects were severely persecuted by state-run religions in both the East and West, simply because their practices posed too great a danger to social norms and established power.

In more than one culture, this secret sexual tradition was called the "left-hand path," while the restrictive, ascetic tradition was called the "right-hand path." This idea is rooted in the archetype that the left is the more passive side of the body, and so is associated with the feminine principle and with sexuality. Because so many people have been indoctrinated into the idea that sexuality is something impure and unspiritual, when left-hand-path practices were discovered from time to time by the brutal hordes of deranged and sexually repressed humanity,

they were quickly branded as evil, without any inquiry into their philosophy and intentions. Many people, throughout history and to this day,
simply consider sex magick to be dirty black magick, something conducted by unchaste libertines specifically to exploit sexual partners and
satiate perverted desires under the thin veil of something spiritual. In
some cases, this is true—especially today, when these techniques are as
readily available to the charlatan as to the saint.[3]

Theosophy and the Left-hand Path

The concept of the left-hand path was first introduced to popular
Western culture through the Theosophical Society. Because of the
Society's extremely sexually inhibited founding philosophy, this path—
the *Vama Marga*—was simply identified as one of evil black magick.
H. P. Blavatsky, the society's founder, declared that, " . . . owing to the
final crisis of physiologico-spiritual adjustment of the races, humanity branched off into its two diametrically opposite paths: the right- and
the left-hand paths of knowledge or of Vidya. Thus were the germs
of the White and the Black Magic sown in those days."[4] Blavatsky
seeks, throughout her writings, to identify the brothers of the left-
hand path as purveyors of the wickedness of every age. "The Bible,"
she argues, "from Genesis to Revelations, is but a series of historical
records of the great struggle between white and black Magic, between
the Adepts of the right path, the Prophets, and those of the left, the
Levites, the clergy of the brutal masses."[5] In fact, the opposite is a more
accurate depiction.

   Ironically, the next author to apply this term to evil magicians was
Aleister Crowley, probably the most famous libertine and sexual Gnostic
of all time, and one who was often accused of being a black magician
himself. He certainly adopted the phrase left-hand path into his own
mythos directly from Blavatsky's writings, probably without any idea of
its sexual connotation. He firmly identified himself as a right-hand-
path master throughout his life. Had he been aware that the real deri-
vation of the phrase came from sexual Tantra, I sincerely doubt that he
would have written as he did about it. Had he realized that the left-
hand path was the sexual path, the libertine path designed to blast
through repression to freedom, he would likely have identified himself as its foremost adept. Instead, he remarks, "These are they who 'shut
themselves up,' who refuse their blood to the Cup, who have trampled
Love in the Race for self-aggrandizement."[6]

Crowley's view of the left-hand path was that its constituents refused to allow their egos to dissolve in "the Holy Graal, that is the sacred vessel of our Lady the Scarlet Woman, Babalon the Mother of Abominations, the bride of Chaos, that rideth upon our Lord the Beast." [7] This quote is, of course, also a metaphor for the act of sexual magick itself. In order to conduct sex magick properly, you must allow your ego to dissolve totally in orgasmic ecstasy, giving every drop of your consciousness to "Babalon." The same holds true for mystics who seek the highest illumination. Liberation is the complete annihilation of your previous concept of yourself upon the discovery of the transcendent unity of all things in Godhead. According to Crowley, brothers of the left-hand path were adepts who refused to allow the complete annihilation of their lower selves, instead conducting "efforts to insulate and protect [themselves], and to aggrandize [themselves] by predatory practices." [8] He basically identified these "Black Brothers" as anyone who sought to restrict human evolution and freedom, including his personal enemies, most organized religions, and particularly Christianity. "Their false compassion is called compassion," he warns, "and their false understanding is called understanding, for this is their most potent spell."

One can also argue that Crowley's concept of the Black Brothers included those ascetics who renounced sexuality, and that all chaste religious practitioners "refused their blood to the cup." In this view, Crowley has simply reversed the whole concept of right- and left-hand paths. [9] It is ironic and amusing to note that many of Crowley's enemies whom he identified as Black Brothers were, in fact, involved in the same Theosophical Society that provided him with his own erroneous ideas about the phrase. [10]

The phrase "left-hand path" was then further degraded by Anton LaVey, who, having half-read some of Crowley's books, created his own Church of Satan and identified his work with the left-hand path, clearly out of a simple desire to be contrary and naughty. LaVey also elevated the lower desires and the ego to the highest place in the philosophy of his "church," seeking self-aggrandizement for its own sake, and this didn't really have anything in particular to do with Satan.

From its beginnings in the practices of sexual gnosis, the term left-hand path has degenerated into an image of simple ego-inflation and corruption. So, should we, as modern Western sex magicians, attempt to re-embrace this term? Several Western adepts have done just that, at least attempting to reconnect with its Tantric roots. But why intentionally choose to describe yourself with a term that causes so much confusion—

a culturally biased term that serves primarily to intimidate and distract rather than enlighten? Why choose to spend precious time explaining and educating, rather than simply existing and enjoying the bliss of sexual gnosis? True sexual sorcerers, freed from any and all limiting concepts, are of course free to leap from path to path at pleasure!

Sexual Magick and Magical Energy

For good or ill, the pearls have been cast, Pandora's box has been opened, the fruit of the Tree has been eaten, and the secrets of sexual magick have now largely been unveiled to the world. Countless books have been written about it in the last thirty years, revealing its techniques. These books range from mere relationship-enhancement love manuals to bizarre grimoires of erotica. The core sexual techniques common to nearly all of them are, in fact, the outer practices of an inner life of spirituality and self-discovery that is inherently sexual, and innately sacred and magical. But if you view sex-magical practices merely as magick tools, relationship band-aids, or sexual aids, you are headed toward potential disaster, and are certainly not likely to improve either your relationships or your magick. The methods of true sexual magick form the basis of an evolutionary path that explores the sacredness of the physical and reveals the transcendent presence of divine power in the heart of primal carnality.

The idea that sexuality can be used to enhance or launch magical energy is now also frequently mentioned in modern works on the general subject of magick, at least in passing. I have even treated the idea briefly in my previous published works. However, this highly important subject is rarely given much realistic practical attention. In fact, in works that purport to be entirely practical "sex-magick guides," many of the simplest problems that arise in sex workings are not even addressed. Making sex magical can be a complicated and sensitive issue, because so much is at stake in our sex lives. Our feelings are easily hurt in these matters because we all want to feel like accomplished lovers, capable of truly satisfying our partners and bringing ourselves into the pure ecstasy of sexual bliss. But many of us are not even satisfied with our own orgasms, let alone convinced of our ability to please our partners. When we bring magick into the equation, things can get even messier.

Many men have chronic difficulties with premature ejaculation or impotence, and many women, at least sometimes, find it hard to reach orgasm in the sex act at all. All of this makes sex magick and sexual mysticism a potentially overwhelming and scary affair. Many modern books claim sex magick is "fun and easy," but this is rarely true. It is the work of the magical adept; it is powerful and karmic; it quickly reveals your limitations, fears, and taboos. Its practice forces you to confront and understand deep parts of yourself that you may never even have realized existed. This is not always either fun or easy. Of course, it is possible to avoid the risks of self-exploration by simply seeking pleasure and manipulating others with the powers you gain. But this will take you into a terrible place—with which, unfortunately, I am all too familiar.

From my own personal struggles and experiences, I know that it is possible to overcome many of these pitfalls and I have practical experience in dealing with many potential problems that can arise. I also know that magical sex is one of the most beautiful sacraments that you can share with another human being.

Starting Down the Path

It's not easy to begin practicing sex magick. When you use sex magically, you are faced with many obstacles right from the beginning. There is great potential for all kinds of awkwardness when you start transforming your sexuality into something more than just "good, dirty, smutty fun." Sexual magick requires control of your mind and your bodily functions, and a capacity for opening up to forces that are beyond your normal consciousness. You must immediately face your own sexual limits, and any limiting ideas you may have about sex. Even suggesting to your partner that you are interested in exploring sex magick can be embarrassing and intimidating. The ensuing conversation will necessarily be very complex: Why would we want to do that? Is there something wrong with our current sex life? What are we going to use it for?

Sex magick is a very touchy subject and must be handled carefully. Your sex partner may feel that such an extravagance is unnecessary if you are truly satisfied sexually, that you are using it as a fantasy escape from the relationship, and that it will cause distance between you rather than a deeper connection. Your partner may also not be at all interested, and then you must consider how to handle this hurdle as well. My own stumbles down this often murky path have consisted of many falls over painful precipices. Hopefully, I can provide you with a few useful guideposts to smooth your way.

The Myth of Semen Loss

In the secret Eastern literature of sexual occultism there are numerous warnings that the male must preserve the *bindu*, or *ching (jing)*, or *chi*[11] found in semen. This theory occupies many pages in both ancient and modern sexual yoga treatises. I now firmly believe this all stems from a sort of spiritual poverty—a fear somewhere in the male psyche that releasing sperm depletes the body's energy. And this is sometimes true. There are times when orgasm results in feelings of fatigue. But not always; sometimes it is invigorating. And your energy level returns to normal in a short while. If your partner is stimulating enough, you will be ready to have more sex in just a short time. Why should there be any limit on the amount of energy available to you? This energy courses through you all the time, coming in with air, food, water, emotion, sunlight, and every other experience. The energy of the universe is infinite, and this infinity is available to you all the time.

Why is it, then, that men seem to have an innate fear of losing sex fluids? I believe this fear stems from the fact that they lose the rigidity of their erections after sexual intercourse and that it takes varying periods of time before they can achieve erection again. This fear is also linked with the perception that, while men are depleted by orgasm, women are often exhilarated and energized. This perpetuates the idea that something is lost by the male partner and gained by the female partner. This is only in appearance, however. Women give just as much energy in the sex act as men. Sometimes that energy differs in quality, but certainly not in quantity. There is no energetic vampirism going on. If you feel that releasing your semen in orgasm drains you, you will be drained. But if you feel that you are sharing mutual energies in the sex act, and that you are a passageway for infinite energy, then you will be fortified by sex.

There is also a popular myth that the time it takes to become erect again after the sex act increases as a man gets older. This myth reinforces fears about losing virility. At age thirty-two, I can still get an erection within fifteen minutes after a powerful orgasm if I am moved by the desire. The fear of losing sexual potency over time, or with excessive sexual expression, is just a myth whose results are produced by expectation. If men feel they are losing something essential in orgasm, then they do. If they feel that there is an infinite abundance of sexual energy in the universe that they can tap into again and again for as long as they want, then they can experience that too. It took me a long time to come to this realization, and it may take you some time to shake off your own fears.

For practical magick—magick used to obtain material ends—I now almost exclusively use sexual techniques or some combination of sexual magick and one of my New Hermetics tools. This sort of magick requires an expenditure of my semen, but my practical results have been nearly one hundred percent effective for quite a while now, and many of the miracles I have produced have been really surprising. I am careful, however, to use my sexual magick only for purposes that directly relate to the accomplishment of my True Will. We will explore this subject more fully later.

Becoming a Sexual Sorcerer

I call this book *Sexual Sorcery* because a sorcerer is traditionally a solitary magick user, or a magician with informal bonds to a small group of other sorcerers. Sorcerers are not bound by oaths to any mystery school or priesthood, and so freely partake of whatever magical principles and techniques are readily at hand. They take principles from many different schools of thought, applying what is practical from whatever systems and philosophies they encounter. They hunt the universe for power, like beasts in the wilderness, grabbing it whenever it is available. Sometimes sorcerers are viewed as "lower magicians," lacking the formal credentials of the magi, but often this gives them more power and freedom to explore magick in whatever way seems most useful. Sorcerers know many secrets that even the highest initiates don't know, because they are not afraid to or forbidden from trying anything.

By sorcery, I do not mean the use of magick for low or material ends. Sorcerers still ultimately have the highest magical aims—transcendence, illumination, liberation—but their methods always employ whatever is within easy reach. While I have been initiated into numerous occult orders, I generally prefer to approach sex magick from the perspective of a sorcerer, free from the restrictions of an order or guru, so that I can take useful ideas and techniques from wherever seems most appropriate to me in my life. Here, I attempt to present a wide range of tools, ideas, and techniques so that you can decide for yourself what your own sexual sorcery will be. We will explore the heights of mysticism and the spiritual transformations of sexual alchemy, as well as the use of sex magick for accomplishing miracles. Sorcery, after all, is certainly a quest for power, and you will discover the pathway to real magical and sexual power in this volume.

This book contains exercises to help you develop as a sexual sorcerer. They are somewhat different from exercises found in other books. While they are basically progressive, you need not do them in any particular order. You can approach them in any order you find helpful to your development. In fact, many of them are quite basic, and you can feel free to "skip ahead" if you are already familiar with a certain area. In fact, it may be helpful to read through the book once, and then go back to conduct the practical work that suits your needs.

This book is for everybody, both seasoned magicians and novices. If you are relatively unfamiliar with magical practices, you will find a number of useful skill-building exercises. If you are already a veteran of the Lesser Banishing Ritual of the Pentagram and other starting practices, you can probably safely skip some of the earliest practical work. I do suggest that you at least examine these exercises, however, as there may be something useful that you've never thought of before, even in the most basic ones. Some of the exercises in this book require a willing and open partner. If you do not have a partner at this time, don't let this discourage you. Simply skip over these exercises until you have found a sex-magical partner.

A Magical Journal

I strongly suggest that you record all of your magical experiences in some sort of journal. If you keep a journal already, good for you. If not, please start keeping one today. Go out and buy a blank notebook, and begin recording your results in as much detail as you care to. Your journal need not be an elaborate leather-bound tome. Any simple spiral-bound notebook will do just fine. Write down your practices, as well as any thoughts, observations, or insights that come up. Any random thought is worthy of recording if it seems interesting to you. Start to keep a real record of your thoughts. Much of this book began as random thoughts in my own journal.

Also, begin to record your dreams when you remember them. This is of great practical importance, as many magical and mystical insights come to you in the form of dreams. Many archetypal forces in your life make their presence known in your nocturnal journeys, and these are of primary importance in your development. Your dream life also often plays out sexual themes, both directly and symbolically, and you will find rich ore for contemplation and understanding of yourself in your dreams. Keep your journal by your bed at night and record what-

Pp. 13-14

ever you remember in th   nly remember a few images, write them dowr   onscious will recognize that you want access   ou will recall things more and more vividly.

The Magical Mirror of the Self

Another way to prepare yourself to become a sexual sorcerer is to truly get to know your inner self. Try removing all of your clothing and standing naked, without makeup or jewelry, by yourself, in front of a full-length mirror.

1. As you look at yourself, without any mask or covering, what are your first impressions?
2. How do you feel about yourself honestly?
3. How do you feel about your body?
4. How do you feel in your body right now?
5. Are there places in your body that hold tension, anxiety, fear?
6. Are there places in your body where you feel pleasure, contentment, joy?
7. How do you feel emotionally overall?
8. Standing before you in the mirror is the person you seek to make an avatar of sexual divinity. Are you worthy?
9. What do you love about yourself?
10. What do you wish you could change about yourself?

Write down all of your impressions in your journal. They will become the raw material in the alchemical operation you are about to commence. This is the base substance that you will transform into gold. Make every effort to regard yourself with the greatest love from this moment on. If you have seen things you do not like in the mirror, understand that these are shadows that will pass. You are a beautiful being of light, and all fulfillment and happiness will come to you in time. If you have seen things that you adore in the mirror, continue to adore them, but remember that humility is also requisite for the true sexual sorcerer.

Become Self-aware

Try to spend the next week becoming conscious, at least for a few minutes at every opportunity that presents itself, of how you feel in different circumstances of life. As you walk down the street, as you sit in traffic, as you engage in work, as you socialize, what emotions do you feel? Take note of both positive and negative emotions and note them in your journal. This information will be of critical importance later in your work.

Discover what makes you uncomfortable, what makes you happy, what scares you, what triggers emotional pain, what brings you ecstasy. Find out what brings you the greatest happiness in your life, and what causes you the most pain. By learning these habitual emotional patterns, you begin to understand your challenges and your strengths on the road ahead. You begin to understand what has scarred you, and what you are really seeking out of your experience in the world. This will help you discover your True Will—your destiny—and the impediments between you and its accomplishment more surely than perhaps any other activity.

Know Your Sexual Self

A useful way to start this process of discovery is to write down your thoughts about your own personal sexuality in your magical journal. This helps you think consciously about your sexuality and your sexual needs. Try answering the following questions and feel free to add any and all additional information that comes to mind. If you are currently in a relationship, it may be helpful to discuss some of these questions with your partner, but don't feel compelled to share them all.

1. What do you think of sexuality generally?
2. What do you think of your sexuality?
3. How would you rate your current sexual experiences?
4. Do you feel satisfied by your sexuality?
5. How would you rate your sex drive right now?
6. Do you feel that you have a stronger or a weaker drive toward sex than your current or recent partners?
7. What are the specific things that turn you on with a sexual partner?
8. What are the specific things that turn you off with a sexual partner?
9. Do you find your sexual interest diminishes with the same partner over time? Describe your experiences in detail.
10. How often do you masturbate? How do you masturbate and what do you think about?

11. Describe your orgasms, both with partners and by yourself, in as much detail as you can—physiologically, psychologically, and spiritually. Are you completely satisfied by your orgasms?

12. Do you feel there is a difference between your orgasms with a partner and those you have when masturbating? If so, describe this for yourself.

13. Do you feel that your sex partners are generally trying to meet your needs during sex?

14. How could your needs be better met?

This book is for anyone interested in developing the ultimate frontiers of their sexual vistas. Throughout, I speak in mostly heterosexual terms, but I believe that the same basic techniques can easily be applied to homosexual relations as well. I have simply never explored homosexual magick, so it would really be rather presumptuous of me to write much about it. However, you must always keep in mind that sex magick, although capable of bringing you to great heights of pleasure and ecstatic union, is not necessarily always good for relationships, nor is it just great sex. It is an initiatory adventure into yourself and your connection to the sexual archetypes within you. This adventure may be very troubling to the status quo, exposing limitations, inflicting trauma, and dredging up pain from all that you have experienced in life. As your unconscious becomes conscious, you discover both your weaknesses and your strengths. The alchemical fire of love fuels this process, slowly burning away the dross and exposing the true philosophical gold. Through the interplay of these unconscious forces, you can discover your true self and your true destiny. If you are ready, this adventure now awaits you.

CHAPTER 1

Sex Magick in Western Civilization

Tear down that lying spectre of the centuries: veil not your vices in virtuous words: these vices are my service; ye do well, & I will reward you here and hereafter.

—Liber AL vel Legis, I, 61

Now, for the great revelation. We Americans are practically all libertine sexual sorcerers already, and really have been since at least the early 1900s. As a culture, we seek pleasure almost exclusively in worldly things; our interests are primarily in sex, physical possessions, and our own personal pleasure and instant gratification. Traditional "spiritual values" have all but disappeared. This cultural shift has taken on an ugly overtone, but, in its essence, it contains many of the ideals of libertine Gnosticism. It only lacks the element of the sacred and transcendent.

We are all obsessed with the baseness all around us. It is fed to us through the television, the Internet, magazines, and movies. We consume it through promiscuous sex, masturbation, drugs (whether pharmaceutical, over-the-counter, or illegal), cigarettes, alcohol, food, and shopping. Whether we drink too frequently, cannot resist a good sale, constantly allow ourselves to get into strange sexual circumstances, download gigabytes of porn daily, or secretly can't miss a single episode of "Oprah," we are all obsessed with the baseness of the mundane world. Whether we partake of it secretly or openly, the mundane is at the center of most people's lives. But the secret to sexual Gnosticism is to see the sacred in the mundane, to identify as holy the very things that the world holds up as sinful. When we sanctify the base things that we so secretly adore with "true love," we make them holy. Thus each connection, each soap opera, each anal sex encounter or bong hit becomes a connection with Godhead. This is the magick of active experience—through active interaction with the lower parts of nature in order to find God present even there. And the key to this is, of course, love.

This is the sexual sorcerer's alchemical secret—the art of transforming baseness into holiness. By offering your true love to what is considered dirty and sinful, your interaction with the mundane world becomes an interaction with holiness, and you are raised to the kingdom of heaven from within the physical world. Ancient civilizations recognized the sacredness of all things, and saw divinity in many places currently considered "naughty." There were gods of sex, love, wine, death, and war. But these gods slowly fell into disfavor as their areas of power became more and more taboo within societies.

You can raise up these ancient powers through love. But this loving adoration must be conducted under the direction of your will. You must choose what you will raise in this way according to how it will benefit you in your life's goals. True love must only be given to things that will aid, or at least not hinder, your True Will. It is of no use to sleep with gossiping street hookers if it is your destiny to be the president of the United States. Instead, it would be wiser to sleep with politicians' daughters, or at least girls who go to Yale.

To me, romantic love is the epitome of experiences that can be sanctified, but perhaps that is just my artistic soul. In any case, your choices must be made in the light of your true destiny, and you can only discover your true destiny by looking within.

Since you are reading a book called *Sexual Sorcery*, you are most likely interested in practicing this Gnostic sanctification of the mundane through sexuality. To begin the process, you must equilibrate your passions generally, so that you consciously choose pathways that are helpful to you. You can only approach the sanctification of the sex force in your life when you have a thorough knowledge of your true nature. You must explore yourself and discover your imbalances, so that you can choose which imbalances ultimately help and which hurt you. This is an evolutionary process. The universe evolves through an interplay of balance and imbalance. In your own development, conscious imbalance leads to new equilibrium on a higher level in an ever-expanding pattern of equilibrium and imbalance, which in turn leads to ultimate Godhead. Once you have learned how to transcend into the divine through wisely chosen vices, you can connect directly to the center of your power, your inner link with the cosmic Logos and Sophia. Then what you project into this center will come to pass.

Your sexual magick is sanctified by your direct connection with the divinity within sex. If you have clearly understood all of this, the rest of this book is unnecessary. All you need to do is go forth and you will be the most powerful sexual sorcerer in the world. But this is all easier said than done. Most of us are far too repressed and neurotic to approach this work without a great deal of preliminary work. Hopefully, this book will help you to succeed.

A Brief History of Sacred Sex

Modern sex-magical treatises invariably begin with a long, and perhaps irrelevant, historical survey of sexual practices around the world. We are, after all, not living in Mesopotamia, so the practices and beliefs of the Sumerians or Babylonians have only a marginal value for us. The sacredness and sanctity of sex and sexual deities is a distant memory, replaced almost entirely, in our society, by the new gods of latex MILFs, penis enlargement formulas, squirting teens, and Viagra. There is, of course, a potential for sacredness even in these images,[12] but they are a far cry from the stone temples of sacred sexuality that were centers of worship all over the world in millennia long past. Still, it is useful to examine, at least briefly, the origins of the traditions we will discuss here, with an eye toward the mythological basis of sacred sex.

It is impossible to trace a clear pathway of sexual practices from one master to the next—particularly in the West—or even from one secret organization to its next incarnation. Sexual religion has often been a secretive endeavor, even in its earliest forms. The secrets of transmuting the base sexual impulse into the gold of enlightenment and magical power have always been reserved for the few. Because of this, these practices have only come to light when discovered by the horrified, repressed masses, who garbled their beauty and power into perversion or nonsense. They are often, therefore, swiftly crushed once discovered. However, these secrets are imperishable, and when one branch of the sacred tree of sexual knowledge withers or is cut, another sprouts—whether through direct secret transmission or spontaneous inspiration, it is impossible to know for certain.

The methodology, philosophy, and technology of this tradition is consistent, however, in nearly all of its manifestations, through all of its iterations, and under all of its names and guises. We can generally consider it one phenomenon. Its initiates may or may not have known each other, and they may or may not claim a common source. In this book, although I will touch upon Eastern sexual mysticism in several places, I will focus primarily on the Western traditions of practical sex magick. Our practical approach to the sex mysteries will necessarily be eclectic, however, since many Eastern ideas have been incorporated into Western magick and mysticism for hundreds of years. In fact, many writers and magicians assert that Western sexual practices, if they ever really had a tradition, are merely a fractured legacy with no clear lineage or history, and that modern practices have largely been pieced together from the traditions of Tantra and other Eastern magical and mystical schools.

Adding to this confusion, many of the early modern proponents of sexual magick in the West, including Paschal Beverly Randolph, Karl Kellner, and Theodore Reuss, claimed a dubious Eastern source for their work in a time when all that was "oriental" seemed wise and exotic. Truthfully, we still live in that time, as yoga, Buddhism, and a hundred other Eastern philosophies still retain a stronghold on the Western mind.

There are, however, several components of sex magick that are distinctly Western—components that come from the unique cultural heritage of the West and are expressed in terms peculiar to it. The lineage of these teachings, if there is one, is highly unclear, particularly through the Middle Ages into the twentieth century. Oaths of secrecy, persecution by the Church, and obfuscation by its proponents and their imitators have rendered the history of Western sex magick blurry at best. We can, however, establish the mythological constructs that underlie its sexual gnosis.

ANCIENT SEX TRADITIONS

The urge to connect sex, religion, and magick has existed through all times—among European pagans, as well as the Greeks, Egyptians, and Romans. Sacred prostitution existed in most ancient Mediterranean, North African, and Middle Eastern civilizations. Women who participated in these rites were considered representatives, avatars, goddesses in the flesh. There was even a tradition in some Mesopotamian cultures that every woman had to go to the temple at least once in her life and act as an avatar of the goddess for the first man who approached her.

To have sex with one of these priestesses was to make love to the goddess herself. Men went to them for all of the usual magical reasons: increased wealth, good luck, to obtain love, for favor from the Goddess of Love, or to exact revenge upon an enemy. Some went simply to worship the divine feminine. Kings were often assigned the task of making love to a goddess through a sacred priestess to assure her continued favor on the society over which he ruled, and to grant authority from the goddess to his rulership.

This practice was pervasive and was not formally stopped until Christian orthodoxy took hold across the ancient world. Wherever orthodox Christianity flourished, the priestesses were transformed quickly into degenerate whores, and the goddesses cast into the darkness of the pit. These cast-out goddesses stubbornly re-emerged right into the middle of the Christian Church, however, as Mary the virgin mother, Magdalene the reformed whore, and even the whore of Babylon, mother of all abominations, whose description seems very similar to a number of Middle Eastern goddesses such as Astarte, Inanna, and Ishtar. Refusing to be supplanted, they were forced to wear new garments that severely limited their role in society. Sexuality came to be viewed as evil, and no sexually positive female image was allowed to remain.

SEXUAL GNOSTICISM

In the earliest forms of Christianity, it was not enough simply to accept Christ as your personal savior in order to obtain salvation. There was some actual spiritual work involved in the original religion. The primitive idea of salvation was something specific, not the vague metaphysical muddle of today's Christianity. To be saved meant that, instead of going to Hades, the traditional land of the dead, when you died, you rose into the heavens to be among the immortal beings—angels, daimons, God. You became part of the divine world. What's more, you could achieve this before death by raising your spirit into the eternal world through various practices, thus making you free from all sin and error—in short, a divine being in the flesh. In modern terms, you raised your energetic vibrations to a higher level than the rest of humanity.

This elevation, this enlightenment, gave you access to greater resources. You might be given the gift of prophecy, or begin to speak in tongues; you might acquire the power to heal or to raise the dead. These powers were granted by the Holy Spirit to those who conducted themselves in accord with certain behaviors and practices. Most of these practices have now been lost, but hints to some of them remain in the fragments of Gnostic Christian scripture, and even in the Bible—at least in the form of behavioral taboos that led you to this divine state.

It is among Gnostic Christians that we find most of the practical advice about how to obtain spiritual gifts and rise up into the divine. There were many incantations and meditative practices designed to lead you to and guide you within higher planes, although all are now lost to modern Christianity. There were also many extended magical operations for obtaining love or sex, and even ones designed to avenge a scornful lover. It is hard to determine which of these practices related to the teachings of Jesus and which were simply pieces of older religion grafted onto the Christian mythos, although it is clear that at least some were part of the pearls that Jesus warned should not be "cast before the swine." Jesus, if there ever really was such a being, was clearly initiating his pupils into something mystical—something that did not make it into the Bible in its completed form.

As Christianity developed, many different belief systems formed within its greater structure. Each viewed its teachings as correct, and the others as "heretical." Christianity today is simply an aggregation of those schools of thought that managed to wipe out all the others. Quite a few of these divergent streams, these "Gnostic heresies," performed sacred sexual rites. Among them were the Barbelo-Gnostics, the Ophites, the Sethians, and the Simonians. Many anti-Gnostic diatribes by early Church Fathers describe sexual deviance as common among the various heretical sects. "Some of his [the Gnostic teacher Marcus's] disciples, too, addicting themselves to the same practices, have deceived many silly women, and defiled them."[13]

In his strange but fascinating essay, *The Eucharist,* Clement de Saint-Marcq asserts that these sexual mystics were the true Christians, and that the "body and blood of Christ" eaten by the apostles was none other than Christ's sperm. By eating Christ's sperm, the Apostles attained an identity with Christ that set them above the rest of humanity. By extension, those who ate the sperm of someone who ate Christ's sperm, or the sperm of someone who ate the sperm of someone who ate Christ's sperm, were also raised. In other words, the apostolic succession is based upon the sacred consumption of sexual fluids going back directly to Christ, through his sanctified sperm. Saint-Marcq further asserts that this is still the hidden mystery of the Catholic Church, and that the anti-sexual polemics of the Church Fathers, as well as the comments of St. Paul, were veils to protect the true secrets from the unworthy. The Catholic Mass, according to Saint-Marcq, was and is simply an empty mask to conceal the sexual mysteries for the exclusive use of the priests. Certainly the "Agape Feasts" of the earliest Christians were sexual reveries in at least some cases.

There seem to have been two separate, but interrelated, kinds of sexual Gnostic practices described in the reports of the Church Fathers. The first was that some Gnostics, including the Simonians and the Sethians, believed that, since they were "pure beings of light," they were not accountable for their actions on the physical plane. Since they existed on a plane above the rest of humanity, what might be sinful for others was not sinful for them. They consequently felt free to engage in sex and adultery at their leisure, fearing no divine reprisal. They believed themselves to be divine, so all of their acts were divine as well. The second set of sexual practices referred to by the Church Fathers was simply the direct use of sex for spiritual purposes—the type of practices we will discuss throughout this book. In these practices, sexuality was used as an avenue to spiritual experience, and sexual fluids were used as a Eucharist for magical purposes.

There is also some fragmentary evidence of sex practice in the Gnostic Gospels themselves, which leads one to believe that these were not simply false accusations by the Church Fathers, but actual practices conducted by people who felt they were doing something holy. There were Christian sexual mysteries, and the Christians who celebrated them believed that Jesus Christ was a teacher of sexual religious practices. These practices were thus accepted as the correct way for Christians to behave. Sexual magick, necromantic sexual magick, and libertine orgiastic behaviors are clearly described. How much of this was actually happening is impossible to determine, because most of the evidence is found only in the words of the critics of these sexual Gnostics, who, after all, may have been attempting to hide their own sexual practices.

There is a great deal of similarity between the practices attributed to the Gnostics and the practices of the left-hand-path Tantric yogis. Combining sorcery with religion, involving spirits of the dead, graveyard images, taboo-breaking, indiscriminate sacred sexual liaisons within a ritual context between unlikely partners such as sisters and brothers, mothers and sons, fathers and daughters—these are all common to both the ancient sexual gnosis and the Vama Marg (left-hand) Tantra. There is also a good deal of similarity between the metaphysical foundations of many Gnostic sects and the Shaivite and Tantric concepts of the origin of reality. I have seen it suggested in a few places that the Gnostics may have borrowed some of their ideas from the Tantrics, but it seems more likely that both find their source in an unknown, more ancient mystery religion. It may also be that these ideas spring directly from consciousness itself, and that the similarities are based on the fact that we are all human beings, with human spiritual needs and human fantasies—both hideous and sublime.

A careful reading of Paul's epistles shows that many within the "orthodox" early Church had a libertine sexual attitude that Paul felt a strong need to squelch. Sacred sexuality was clearly "epidemic" at this time. "It is reported commonly that there is fornication among you, and such fornication as is not so much as named among the Gentiles, that one should have his father's wife" (I Corinthians 5:1). Of course, this may be another attempt to conceal the sexual mysteries that Paul himself practiced.

It is impossible to know whether this Gnostic, sexualized Christianity was the "real" Christianity, or whether it was simply a combination of older mystery practices with a new Christian flavor. It certainly existed, however, and may not have been entirely squashed by the Church Fathers or even the later council of Nicea, which clearly defined once and for all the doctrine that the Church would uphold. This concrete doctrine was explicitly anti-sexual and anti-life, preferring to direct the attention of the faithful to Christ's death and the promise of ascent into a distant heaven in the far future.

FROM THE MIDDLE AGES TO THE RENAISSANCE

Even with the extreme repression of the Roman Church as it grew to dominate the Western world, Gnostic heresies persisted. Though often threatened with extinction, they merely reappeared in different places in slightly different raiment. Even within the Church itself, mystics like St. Theresa experienced ecstatic visions that could only be described as sexual reveries. These mystics were tolerated, but certainly not encouraged. Heresy was a persistent problem, because genuine spiritual experience always tears through the rules of any religion in which it occurs. Spirituality and organized religion can usually, at best, live side by side, but they rarely share the same bed. The Roman Church did its best to discourage all but the very simplest forms of adherence to its tenets.

Some years after most of the Gnostics had been wiped out, Europe's monarchs, working with the Church, began to spread their influence ever further, attempting to hold back the growing tide of the new upstart religion, Islam. During the Crusades against the Muslims in Jerusalem, the Order of the Knights of the Temple was formed. These Knights quickly became rich, powerful, and influential, much to the dismay of the Church and the royalty of Europe. Rumors began to circulate that they had strange initiatory rites, and that they may have consorted with the Muslims and learned sorcery and other evil practices from these "heathens." The Knights Templar were soon accused of heresies similar to those of the Gnostics—deviant sexual practices, including homosexuality, worshipping idols and skulls of the dead, and black magical practices. It is believed by many that the Knights Templar were initiated by Muslim mystics into secret magical and religious practices, including worship of a generative god called Baphomet. This may also have included certain Gnostic practices and beliefs that had survived Christian persecution. The Templars were disbanded and their leaders burned at the stake.

Soon, fears of a witch cult swept across Europe, and these "witches" were again suspected of practices similar to those of the Gnostics and the Templars. They were accused of sexual deviance, worship of generative gods or simply of Satan, and numerous magical practices. Reports of the medieval witch trials frequently describe the rape of young witches by the ice-cold phallus of Satan. On the whole, these accusations were similar to those lodged against all heretics. Is this because there was a common thread of belief among these groups? Or was there simply a common fear among their accusers? It is impossible to say with any certainty. The similarities, however, indicate that, under the surface of culture, sexual mysteries and magick loomed as a threat and a temptation throughout the Middle Ages. Indeed, the Cathar and Bogomil Gnostic heretics were accused of similar deviant behaviors, although these accusations carry less credence, since the tenets of both of these sects seem asexual, although this may have been an outer veil to conceal the sexual mysteries within.

Esoteric sexual practices are found among a number of Jewish sects as well. Among some, for instance, sexual relations on the eve of the Sabbath are said to assist God in the continuation of the universe, and shine favor down upon the nation of Israel. God is thought to connect with his consort, the Shekinah, or divine presence, on the Sabbath night, and this grace is bestowed upon the universe through the sexual intercourse of the faithful.

In the early fifteenth century, the Rosicrucian manifestos were published anonymously. Their appearance revived interest in the occult.

Many occult scholars believe that the true secrets of the Rosicrucians were sexual mysteries, although no hard evidence of this has ever come to light. Certainly the "third" Rosicrucian manifesto, *The Chymical Wedding of Christian Rosenkreutz,* contains many subtle sexual references. The book is divided into seven chapters, and then subdivided into seven sections in numerous places throughout the text. In fact, the number seven seems to have great significance throughout the book. Seven is the number sacred to Venus, the Goddess of Love, a fact of which the author of the book was most certainly aware.

Venus plays a pivotal role in the allegory of the *Chymical Wedding,* though she is hidden away in the darkness of a basement throughout. One could even say that Venus is the whole hidden power of the book, and love its secret message. At the beginning of the allegory, all impure people are forced to leave, but those who remain, the pure, seem to talk quite a lot about sex. The author of the story clearly does not think sexual thoughts impure. Certainly the love poem of the nymphs is a fairly clear exposition on the author's thoughts on this. Moreover, there is a scene just before the song of the nymphs that is very similar to a traditional Tantric ceremony, in which male and female couples are paired by chance. However, the sexual liaison is prevented by a clever trick that, once again, incorporates the number seven. It is almost certain that the author of the *Chymical Wedding* was imparting something sexual beneath the surface of his tale to those who could understand it. The Formula of the Rosy Cross is a popular veil for sexual magick that we will explore in the coming pages.

Numerous Hermetic, Platonic, and Neoplatonic texts were translated into the vernacular around this time, and a great interest in the esoteric was reborn. Alchemical writings abounded, often incorporating a great deal of sexual imagery into their symbols. Eventually, the Freemason movement appeared out of the darkness, claiming to be a legacy from nearly all of these past heretical groups, while somehow whitewashing their unsavory reputations. According to some, the Freemasons' true initiatory secrets conceal some of these ancient sexual mysteries in complex symbols and veiled imagery, myths, and allegories. If this is true, it is highly unlikely that many current masons are aware of it.

THE NINETEENTH AND TWENTIETH CENTURIES

In some ways, it is easier to talk about the whole occult movement after the advent of the nineteenth century because we can ascertain the names of many of the major players and access an entire literature that expounds their philosophical thought. In other ways it is quite difficult to determine exactly what was going on, because there were so many occult groups at this time with shared memberships and similar names and practices. The names and "histories" of these groups also seemed to change rather organically over the course of time. Our historical literature on them is incomplete, since much of the secret information was never committed to writing or only recorded in sketchy form.

The modern history of sex magick in continental Europe seems to start in a very unusual place—with a black man in the United States—and at a very unusual time—just as slavery was coming to an end. Paschal Beverly Randolph was an African-American man of mixed heritage. His father, Edmund Randolph, was a white politician and his mother, Flora Beverly, was a black woman about whom little is clearly known. A friend of Abraham Lincoln, Napoleon III, and other prominent figures of his time, Randolph really began the whole modern Western sexual occult movement. Claiming at times to have been initiated by Rosicrucians and by "Ansairetic" adepts, and later claiming to have devised his own system of initiation from his fertile, inspired imagination, Randolph developed an occult system that had a profound influence on the awakening Western occult mind.

To this day, there is a great deal of confusion surrounding the groups that Randolph started or in which he played a part. The H B of L—variously identified as the Hermetic Brotherhood of Luxor, the Hermetic Brothers of Light, or the Hermetic Brotherhood of Light—seems to have adopted his system of sex magick wholesale, or else he adopted theirs. The dates seem to indicate that the former is true, but the exact date of the start of the H B of L is highly questionable itself. Blavatsky claimed that the H B of L was originally responsible for the start of her own Theosophical Society, which places its start at a much earlier date than that supplied by the written record. Of course, Blavatsky later disavowed any connection with the H B of L, which used Randolph's sex-magical system, preferring the purer idea of hidden mahatmas dwelling in the high places of the Himalayan Mountains.

By the late nineteenth century, a German named Karl Kellner surfaced with a system of sexual magick that he, like Randolph and Blavatsky before him, claimed came from Eastern adepts. His system, however, seems to derive largely from Randolph's methods with the addition of a bit of confused material on yoga involving various *chakras* and *vayus* (sacred winds). Kellner created an order called Ordo Templi Orientis, O.T.O., which at first seems to have existed largely in his own mind. He eventually became involved with Theodore Reuss and others who had purchased charters for the fringe Masonic degrees of Memphis and Misraim, and together they launched Ordo Templi Orientis as a genuine phenomenon. Reuss proposed to the world that the O.T.O. possessed the true secrets of the symbols of both Freemasonry and the Catholic Church. These symbols revealed predictably the secrets of sexual magick. Various occultists of the age who were involved, in lesser or greater degree, with the Ordo Templi Orientis include Rudolph Steiner, Papus, Franz Hartmann, and eventually the infamous Aleister Crowley.

Crowley was made the Supreme and Holy King of Great Britain and Ireland, and used the opportunity to introduce his new religious doctrine of *Thelema* into the order's grade system and philosophy. Thelema fit very well with the sexual doctrines of the O.T.O., and it seems that, for a time at least, Crowley made a convert out of Reuss. Papus connected his Gnostic Catholic Church to the O.T.O. and Crowley wrote his own version of a Gnostic Catholic Mass, which Reuss seems to have loved and introduced to the order as a whole. However, there was some sort of schism between Crowley and Reuss in the early 1920s and it is unclear whether Crowley was thrown out of O.T.O., or whether he simply fell out of favor with Reuss. At any rate, shortly before Reuss's death, Crowley proclaimed himself the Outer Head of the Order, and assumed the reins of leadership.

Many disagreed with Crowley's leadership, and the order as a whole seems largely to have fallen apart after this. The nature of the disagreement between Reuss and Crowley is obscure, but this much is clear: Crowley had a great deal of respect for Reuss. He kept to the letter of his oath of secrecy regarding the O.T.O.'s secrets throughout his entire life. Crowley made a habit of attacking anyone who opposed him, and he published the secret rituals of the Golden Dawn only ten years before he joined the O.T.O. If Crowley had been maligned by Reuss, I doubt that he would have written so respectfully of him twenty-five years after his death. Crowley had every opportunity to attack Reuss and, although he attacked nearly every other occult authority of his age, he always held Reuss in the highest regard.

Crowley continued his own Thelemic O.T.O. with or without the support of others, starting lodges in the United States with several of

his disciples. By the time of his death, the only really active Thelemic
O.T.O. lodge in the world was in California, and even Crowley was
uncertain about their activities. However, though the order was relatively
inactive, some small connections between the members seem to have
continued into the 1960s, when Karl Germer, then the closest thing
to a chief of O.T.O., died.

After this, three contenders grappled for control of the almost non-
existent O.T.O.: Grady McMurtry, Kenneth Grant, and Marcello Motta.
All three had only very nebulous claims to power, but, when no pro-
vision is made, the kingdom goes to the warrior with the biggest sword.
Apparently this warrior was Grady McMurtry, because a following
quickly swelled around him and he began actively initiating members
at some point in the late '60s or early '70s. Motta, Grant, and their fol-
lowers and allies have fought with McMurtry and his own successor
both magically and through the legal system for the last few decades.
During that time, however, the O.T.O. has grown into a very successful organization, boasting a membership of many thousands that spans
the globe. The sexual secrets of the O.T.O. are still reserved for its highest initiates, however, and this is a much smaller group of people.

Since Crowley's time, the idea that sexuality can be used for mysticism and magick has become quite popular. In the 1920s and '30s, a
number of other groups emerged practicing a brand of sexual magick
that makes it clear that they derived their techniques directly from the
O.T.O. and Aleister Crowley, or at least from Randolph. Among these
are the moderately well-known magical orders Fraternitatis Saturni
and the G∴B∴G∴. The growing interest in sacred sex in the West,
however, was largely due to the importation of Tantric and Taoist practices from the East.

Recently, numerous secrets of Western sex magick have been
revealed by members of Crowley's and related orders. Modern witchcraft has disclosed its ideas about sex magick, which bear a remarkable
resemblance to Aleister Crowley's instructions on the subject. This is
largely because Gerald Gardner, the author of *Wicca's Great Rite*, took
many of his ideas and texts directly from Crowley. A simple glance at
one passage from Gardner's rite suffices as illustration: "Oh circle of
stars whereof our father is but the younger brother, marvel beyond
imagination, soul of infinite space, before whom time is bewildered
and understanding dark, not unto thee may we attain unless thine image
be love."[14] This is directly lifted from Aleister Crowley's Gnostic Mass.[15]

Your Personal Sexual History

Although many books have been written by authorities about sex magick and sex mysticism over the last decades, few have really explained its true meaning. That is because, to a great extent, this meaning can only be found inside yourself. So now, let's take a look at your own sexual history.

Take out your journal and answer the following questions for yourself in writing. By writing these things down, you will discover amazing truths about yourself, and begin to unlock many of your own secret chambers and sexual hiding places.

Building Your Personal Sexual History

1. What are the earliest sexual thoughts you can remember?
2. At what age did you first become aware of your sexual feelings?
3. Are there any early-life traumas that may have affected your interest in sex, either positively or negatively?
4. How was sexuality initially presented to you? By parents? Friends? In what terms?
5. Were your first impressions of sexuality positive or negative?
6. How did the person or persons who first explained sexuality to you color your impressions of it?
7. Describe your first kiss.
8. Describe your first love.
9. Describe your first experience of sexual intercourse.
10. Make a list of all of your past sexual partners, and assess the effect that these relationships had on you both sexually and emotionally.
11. How else has your sexual history affected your current experiences of sexuality?
12. What are your sexual inhibitions and taboos? What would you never do?
13. What are your fetishes? What would you and do you love to do?

Now, describe your ideal sexual partner in as much detail as you can. Use the following questions as a guide, but add anything and everything else you can think of as well. Do not allow feelings of what you "should" want to influence you. What you really want is all that is important.

Defining Your Ideal Sexual Partner

1. What is your ideal sexual partner like?
2. What does your ideal sexual partner look like?
3. How does your partner treat you?
4. How does your partner talk to you?
5. How does your partner touch you?
6. What does your partner give you?
7. How do past or current sexual partners compare to your ideal?
8. How could your current partner modify his/her behavior to fit more closely with your ideal?

This questionnaire may also provide a useful ground for discussion with your current lover, and may be particularly useful for your own meditation regarding your current relationship. But if you do open a discussion about your ideal, you must take care not to hurt your lover unnecessarily. No one is perfect, and you may endanger your intimacy with your partner if he or she falls short of your ideal. At the same time, you should never allow yourself to feel trapped in a situation that does not meet your needs. If your current lover is not the one you really want to be with, consider your reasons for being in such a relationship. On the other hand, if your lover is fairly close to your ideal, this conversation can be very sexy, and lead to all sorts of wonderful intimacy.

If you are not currently in a relationship, this questionnaire gives you the opportunity to explore what you want in your next relationship. By answering these questions honestly and accurately, you can get a real sense of what you want and what you don't want for the future. In this way, when you meet your ideal person, you will know it. This is a very important exercise and should not be ignored.

CHAPTER 2

Sex-Magical Systems

Nor let the fools mistake love; for there are love and love. There
is the dove, and there is the serpent. Choose ye well!
—*Liber AL vel Legis, I, 57*

As we begin to move from the theoretical to the practical, we must lay
down the specifics of the magical framework in which we will work.
As briefly discussed in the last chapter, there are three magical writers
who left a legacy of sexual instruction upon which we can build the edi-
fice of our own sexual awakening. In this chapter, I will describe these
systems in more detail, as well as a few other ideas that will inform our
work. There are, of course, other sexual writers and thinkers who have
greatly influenced esoteric ideas about sexuality, but these three seem
to be the only ones interested in presenting an explicit system of sex
magick, and presenting it in a semi-public manner. We will draw material from all three of these systems, and explore the practical fruits of each,
discovering our own secrets of sexual magick along the way.

Paschal Beverly Randolph and the
Hermetic Brotherhood of Luxor

The modern history of practical sex magick begins with Paschal Beverly
Randolph and the related teachings of the Hermetic Brotherhood of
Luxor, which share virtually identical sex-magical systems. Together,
they were the first to expound sex-magical mysteries to the European
middle class. Randolph left a fairly detailed set of magical instructions,

beginning with directions for the totally untrained neophyte and leading to sexual adepthood. The instructions of the Brotherhood are very
similar to Randolph's, but I will stick with Randolph's descriptions
because they are simpler and less confusing, though sometimes his terminology is a bit odd.

Randolph's system asks novices to develop four distinct abilities
that he called Volantia, Decretism, Posism, and Tirauclairism. These same
basic ideas are found in the instructions of the Brotherhood, which
blended them together and renamed them Formulation, Vitalization, and
Realization.

VOLANTIA

In Randolph's system, Volantia means a calm and focused direction of
the will. The methods both he and the Brotherhood prescribe for the
development of this will are identical. Take a disc of black paper and
attach it to a white wall. Stare at this disc fixedly for a minute or two,
and then look at a blank white surface. An afterimage of the disc will
appear before your eyes. Attempt to hold onto this image for as long
as possible. It will disappear and reappear a few times, but hold onto it
for as long as possible. Later, you can use colored discs to see complementary colors in the afterimage, or even attach a white disc to the
surface of a magick mirror to obtain a similar effect. In theory, this
develops attention, concentration, and the force of attraction. Randolph
makes clear that, if you experience discomfort or fear during these
exercises, you should abandon the path of magick altogether.

According to Randolph, after several months of repeating this exercise for a few minutes each day, you will be able to create any astral
form easily while staring at a white surface, and to communicate with
the forms you create. Luckily, there are less tedious ways to develop
this ability, but this one may be useful to some. You can certainly use
it if all else fails.

DECRETISM

Decretism is the ability to give orders that are instantly obeyed by both
yourself and others. This is not a skill you acquire through exercise, but
rather one that develops on its own—primarily from the disciplined
exploration of the previous practice, but also simply through the course
of a decisive life.

POSISM

Posism is Randolph's system of gestures. It consists of an array of strange postures, movements, and positions that represent and enable various purposes. Decretism gives these poses their power. These poses do not really relate actively to sex magick and would take us quite far afield from our topic. I therefore refer the curious reader to Randolph's work for a clear exposition of this subject.[16] The important point for us here is that, by adopting gestural poses regularly, you imbue them with volitional power.

TIRAUCLAIRISM

Tirauclairism is Randolph's term for the ability to evoke communication with invisible beings like angels, spirits, or the dead. His instructions for developing this ability are very simple. First, master the Volantia exercise. Then simply fix the image of a flaming star in your mind's eye and invoke the desired personal and character traits you want to manifest in yourself through the medium of this flaming star. Invoke qualities that will help you to be a greater being—balanced and powerful. Once you've thoroughly mastered yourself by invoking positive and constructive qualities that balance your passions, you can go on to invoke planetary and celestial qualities, beings, and hierarchies with this same "flaming star" technique. This technique can be used in the midst of or after the sexual act, or even without the use of sex. In fact, Randolph's actual sexual instructions make absolutely no mention of any of these four items ever again.

PRACTICAL SEX MAGICK

Once you have developed the four powers described above, you can begin to explore Randolph's actual system of sex magick. Randolph offers no detailed instruction about sexual techniques or ceremonies. Instead, he confines himself primarily to moral and behavioral instructions for your sexual life. There are really just two basic principles in his instructions: The sex act should be a loving and spiritual connection with someone that you love, and you can accomplish what you want to magically by simply thinking about it throughout the sex act.

Randolph also offers a complex and confusing scheme of mathematical and sometimes arbitrary instructions regarding astrology, perfumes, psychotropic drug stimulants, and fluid condensers that are really far too complex to be practical. I think these instructions may actually represent an attempt to protect the core of magical truth from the unworthy. The essence of sex magick is much simpler.

The sum and substance of Randolph's system is epitomized in the quote that opens this book: "If a man ardently wishes a force or power into being and guards this wish from the instant that he penetrates into the woman until the instant that he withdraws from her, his wish is necessarily fulfilled." What could be simpler? In fact, this is really the essence of all of Western sex magick, summarized simply and concisely in a single sentence. Clearly, Randolph felt that a woman could tap into this power as well. He just uses the sexist vocabulary of his time to convey his point, adding: "It is not said that woman has not the power to assume the initiative in magical operations."

Randolph's view in this regard is actually very important, because most other texts about sex magick really delegate the woman to the role of a tool for the male magician. This, of course, is ridiculous. Women are often more powerful sex magicians than men, and it is interesting to note that the earliest sex-magical instructions are egalitarian and not gender-biased. It is only with Aleister Crowley that sex-magical instructions become sexist.

Randolph's actual instructions for sex magick are extremely simple, though he adds additional instructions to his first formulae that greatly confuse the matter, expanding it into a complicated scheme that takes forty-eight days to accomplish. Ignoring these complications, here are Randolph's basic instructions:

1. Think through your magical purpose in advance, and keep clear images of your goal in your mind throughout the sex act. (This is why you spent all that time staring at discs of paper.)
2. Consider sex as a prayer. Regard whatever you are willing into existence prayerfully throughout the sex act. Both sexual partners should think prayerfully about the same thing.
3. Cleanse all lust from your sex act, and make it a spiritual uniting of your two innermost selves.
4. A female should "tremble with desire" (orgasm?) at least twice before her male partner climaxes.
5. Be sure to think of your magical purpose at orgasm.
6. Your sexual partner should be a worthy one—your lover or spouse, or someone to whom you are devoted—not a prostitute or base person.

7. Keep your intentions secret and private between you and your partner.
8. Be cleanly in your person and in your life.
9. Always eat natural foods and avoid hard spirits (liquor).
10. Sleep and perform your sexual magick on a hard bed with your head oriented to the north.
11. Sleep in a room apart from your partner and only come together once or twice a week for sex.
12. Don't have sex when angry or lustful.

Randolph also describes several sexual positions for various magical purposes that are quite interesting and unique to his writing. These positions are, I suppose, the explicitly sexual version of his Posism. Figure 2 illustrates these positions and the purposes for which you can use them. You can incorporate these positions into your own practical work, though we won't discuss them explicitly.

According to Randolph, you can accomplish the following magical effects with sex magick:

Charging a "volt"[17]
Regenerating personal vitality and magnetism
Producing magnetism to influence or control your sexual partner
Refining your power or senses
Determining the sex of a child
Obtaining visions of higher planes
Gaining success in some project or financial affair

To Randolph's rather tidy little sex system, the Brotherhood of Luxor added a whole cosmological doctrine of world ages that seems derivative of the Theosophical Society's materials. In places, this doctrine is clearly just a politically motivated refutation of some of the society's doctrines—that of reincarnation, for example. These instructions may be useful to some, but have little to do with our subject.[18]

Aleister Crowley, the O.T.O., and the A∴A∴

Crowley is certainly the most famous sex magician of the modern era, though his sex magick is not even particularly well-known in comparison with his reputation as the "bad boy" of occultism. Most people simply view him as a black magician, a Satanist, or as the prophet of the New Aeon of Thelema and Ra Hoor Khuit.

Male Directed   Female Directed

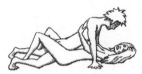   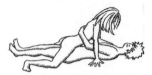

POSITION #1—For correcting senses and invoking desired qualities

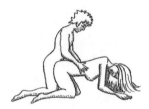   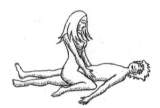

POSITION #2—For projection and influence, charging volts, or creating elementals.

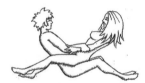   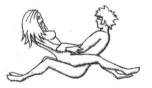

POSITION #3—For invocation as well as for projection and influence

POSITION #4—For harmonizing natures of lovers and for mystical union

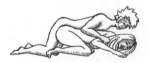   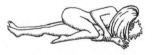

POSITION #5—For secretly influencing your partner or for powerful projection.

Figure 2. Pascal Beverly Randolph's sex positions

It is likely, however, that there would not be a modern magical movement at all without the writings of Aleister Crowley, his students, and his associates. Crowley is the person who coined the term "magick" with a "k." In certain old works, you may see the word spelled this way, but Crowley reintroduced this spelling as standard to the twentieth-century magical revival, and it has been adopted directly through him into the whole neopagan/witchcraft/wicca movement. In truth, even a superficial glance at the revival of witchcraft reveals the incredible debt it owes to Crowley.

It is unfortunate that Crowley is so often derided and vilified within the magical community. If it were not for him and his students, much of the source material for the modern magical movement would still be locked away in dusty libraries and private collections. Gerald Gardner, the father of modern witchcraft, was a student of Crowley's, and the original *Call of the Goddess* contained quite a bit of Crowley material, until Doreen Valiente rewrote it in an attempt to expunge him from the history of witchcraft. The Great Rite of Gardnerian witchcraft is essentially a condensed version of Crowley's Gnostic mass. Some even think that Crowley may have written rituals for Gardner, although even a cursory glance at them shows that this cannot be so. The rituals contain paraphrases of many of Crowley's inspired writings that he would never "change so much as in the style of a letter." The Great Rite uses a paraphrased quote that mixes up the sexual characteristics of the invoked energies in a way that Crowley would never have done. All the same, witchcraft owes much to him.

The term magick with a "k" also has interesting correspondences that relate directly to sex magick. "K" is the eleventh letter of the alphabet, an important magical number that represents the imbalance necessary for any creative act. Balance is stasis. Evolution can occur only in imbalance—change takes place only when the balance shifts away from the center toward one polarity or another and eventually causes a new equilibrium in a more advanced state. So the "k" in magick indicates the imbalance created through the sexual energies that you stir up in your magick, and the changes you precipitate through the use of your will. Crowley supposedly also felt that the "k" was indicative of *kteis,* the female generative organs, secretly indicating that "magick" was the magick of sex.

Crowley's teachings are grounded in the drive toward sexual gnosis through sexual liberation and exploration, though he almost never wrote about sex magick openly. Crowley strongly believed that sex magick, the practice of working magick while engaged in sexual activities, was the great key to all practical magical work. "There is another sacrifice with regard to which the Adepts have always maintained the most profound secrecy. It is the supreme mystery of practical magick. Its name is the Formula of the Rosy Cross."[19] Crowley was bound by oaths of silence to his own magical teacher, Theodore Reuss of the O.T.O., as well as by the laws of Victorian censorship, not to publicly reveal his own explicit techniques for accomplishing sex magick in his published works. I must say, before we go any further, that I have never received any formal training from the O.T.O. in sexual magick, and this book is not in any way a revelation of or an attempt to describe the secrets of the upper degrees of the O.T.O. Although many of the secrets have been described in any number of books, I will not comment specifically on the O.T.O. mysteries. I am an initiate of the O.T.O., but I am not an initiate of its ninth degree and so am not qualified to describe its mysteries in any way. Moreover, I would be restricted by oaths of secrecy from doing so if I were such an initiate. So, when we discuss Crowley's sex magick, please keep in mind that I am describing his work in general terms, not in terms of the work of the O.T.O. specifically.

Sex magick is also an inherent part of the A∴A∴ adept's work. The Formula of the Rosy Cross is one of the main magical formulae of the Adeptus Major in the A∴A∴. Since I have taken numerous oaths to "Proclaim openly my connection with the A∴A∴, speak of It and Its principles (even so little as I understandeth) for that mystery is the enemy of Truth," I feel comfortable discussing Crowley's sexual magick from the perspective of A∴A∴ work.

Crowley referred to sex magick obliquely, veiling its symbolism in vehicles like the Formula of the Rosy Cross throughout his voluminous writings over the course of his life. In fact, once you realize that a vast amount of Crowley's work secretly conceals his instructions in sex magick, a whole new layer of understanding emerges in his dense writing. We will return often to Crowley's obliquely written instructions to understand his sex magick more clearly.

Below are some of the mystical/alchemical words used by Crowley to conceal or obscurely describe sex-magical teachings. Keep in mind, however, that Crowley often uses these same words to describe mystical processes that transcend mere physical sexual acts, and sometimes he appears to be describing both at the same time!

Male operator and/or his *lingam*/phallus: lion, king, Sun, gold, beast, *hadit*, wand, rood, lance, cross, point, pyramid, *tau*, fire, *athanor*

Female operator and/or her *yoni/kteis*: eagle, queen, *babalon*, *nuit*, Moon, silver, cup, graal, cup of abominations, rose, circle, water, *cucurbite*

Male sexual fluids: blood of the lion, blood, blood of the saints, dew, serpent, seed, *bindu*, sap of the world ash wonder tree

Female sexual fluids: gluten, gluten of the eagle, menstruum, egg, orphic egg

Combined sexual fluids: the elixir of life, the elixir, red elixir (when menstrual blood is involved), white elixir (no menstrual blood), the stone of the philosophers, tincture, universal medicine, potable gold, the sacrifice, the male child of perfect innocence and high intelligence, wine of the Sabbath of the adepts, the Eucharist of one element, the sacrament of the gnosis

Sex-magical procedure: Formula of the Rosy Cross, Rosy Cross, *crux ansata* or *ankh*, Sabbath of the adepts, Mass of the Holy Ghost, the chymical marriage or chymical nuptials, mystic marriage, the royal art

The essence of Crowley's sex-magical system is quite similar to Randolph's in a number of ways, and, like Randolph's, it is really quite uncomplicated. Launching a magical wish with your orgasm is the essential element of both systems. "Only in the end shalt thou give up thy sap when the great God F.I.A.T. is enthroned on the day of Be-with-Us."[20] But there are several important differences. Crowley adds a great deal of Qabala and metaphysics to his system. The idea of the Eucharist, using the sexual fluids as a consecrated magical *telesma*, either to be eaten or placed onto a magical object, was very important to Crowley—an idea that does not enter Randolph's writings. In his *magnum opus, Book 4*, Crowley describes the Eucharist of the sexual fluids in this way: "The highest form of Eucharist is that in which the Element consecrated is One. It is One substance and not two, not living and not dead, neither liquid nor solid, neither hot nor cold, neither male nor female."[21] This combining of male and female sexual essences into one substance thus turned into something divine by physical and psychological action, makes up the substance of this Eucharist. Of its virtue, he writes: "It is the Medicine of Metals, the Stone of the Wise, the Potable Gold, the Elixir of Life."[22] Of course, this "god-eating" of sexual fluids is very reminiscent of Gnostic and even Eastern Tantric sex practices.

In Crowley's sex magick, these charged fluids are considered the incarnation of a little magical god that expresses the will of the magician or magicians. Man and woman are incomplete images of the divine by themselves, but when they come together, they represent the totality of existence—male-female, positive-negative, active-passive. The male and female in union encompass all possibilities. So what they create in this connection is something of great potential holiness and power. By raising consciousness to union with the inner divine essence during the sex act, the combined sexual fluids become the divine offspring of a union of gods.[23]

Crowley saw great power in homosexual unions as well—in contrast to Randolph, who mentions nothing but heterosexuality and monogamy. Crowley seemed to revere both homosexuality and promiscuity. He also frequently conducted his sex magick with prostitutes, in direct opposition to Randolph's ideas.

In several places, Crowley indicates that he really believed male homosexual sex magick to be the most powerful formula—more powerful than heterosexual or lesbian acts. "The great merits of this formula are that it avoids contact with the inferior planes, that it is self-sufficient, that it involves no responsibilities, and that it leaves its masters not only stronger in themselves, but wholly free to fulfill their essential natures."[24] Elsewhere, he writes: "O my Son, the Doors of Silver are wide open, and they tempt thee with their Beauty; but by the narrow Portal of Pure Gold shalt thou come more nobly to the Sanctuary."[25]

Crowley also used masturbation in his sex magick, while Randolph made no mention of masturbation at all. It is unclear whether masturbatory sex magick was a part of the early O.T.O. instructions that spawned Crowley's ideas, or whether he added this himself. The few materials I've seen written by Reuss do not indicate anything at all about masturbation, but it may have always been a part of the upper-degree oral instructions.

CROWLEY'S SEX MAGICK

The essence of a Crowley sex-magick operation is fairly simple, and he described them publicly under veils of symbolism in many places in his writings. Crowley wrote a broad outline for sexual operations called the *Grimoirium Sanctissimum*, which he published in *Book 4*. It appeared originally in Latin only, but the newest edition contains a complete English translation.[26] In it, he uses elements from both A∴A∴ and O.T.O. as the "liturgy" of his operation, but you can easily replace his suggestions with words of your own, as he seems to have done on many occasions. The Gnostic Mass is a pantomime of the exact same steps outlined in the *Grimoirum Sanctissimum*. He also describes this same operation in several places in *Liber Aleph*.[27] In fact, this book contains a huge amount of veiled sexual instruction of various sorts. The Star Sapphire conceals this same operation, as does much of his explanatory instruction in *Liber Samekh*. The two papers *Liber Cheth vel Vallum Abiegni* and *Liber A'ash vel Capricorni Pneumatici* describe this same operation in highly symbolic terms. The novel *Moonchild* depicts an extended operation of this sort, in which the participants attempt to incarnate a lunar being physically. There are numerous other places where he reveals at least some portion of this technology.

A typical Crowley sex-magick operation is fairly simple and straightforward. Each of its elements can be found in almost all of the above referenced materials, although the ceremonial aspects appear to be optional. It is important to decide your purpose in advance and all participants must work toward the same purpose in the operation. This purpose must be in sympathy with the True Will of the operators. Sometimes, participants make talismans or collect other ritual objects; sometimes they choose a spirit to embody the work. Preparations include bathing, consecrations, and any initial ceremonial opening rituals, including invocations of god-forms. These do not seem to be essential to the operation, however, as long as the magician(s)[28] raises consciousness, and hence the resulting sex fluids, to a magical place. The whole operation essentially prepares for the incarnation of an omnipotent little god.

Once preparations have been made and opening rituals performed, the participants stimulate each other's genitals until they are aroused, continuing any verbal invocations. While becoming aroused, you can briefly forget the purpose of the operation, so that you can become really passionate.

The sex act then begins, and the mind turns back to the purpose of the operation. The sex must extend for as long as possible; no less than a half an hour. Focus on your purpose as intensely as possible, directing it through the ecstatic connection with your partner. This ecstasy should be very strong, and your effort to focus should be supreme. Continuously visualize that you are preparing the way of incarnation for your force. A mantra, spell, or rhyming incantation can be used to direct your attention.

Continue the sex until you are in pure ecstasy, lost to all but the intensity of what you are doing. Orgasm should be simultaneous with your partner if possible, indicating the singularity of the act. At the moment of orgasm, though the conscious mind is lost in ecstasy, the will must be entirely focused on the operation.

The sexual fluids are then gathered. A portion of them can be placed on the talisman or on the "magical link" if you are using either one or both. The practitioner(s) must consume the rest by placing the fluids under the tongue, to be absorbed directly into the membranes.

This is basically the whole of Crowley's A∴A∴ sex-magical technology, at least from his publicly available writings. There are a couple of unpublished pieces that I have never seen, but I doubt they offer much more than what you see here. However, this outline leaves aside a number of metaphysical elements that we will explore a little more fully in the next chapter.

In *De Arte Magica*,[29] Crowley suggests ten different purposes suitable to sex-magick operations. He ties them to the ten sephiroth of the Tree of Life:

1. To increase your personal sex force and powers of sex attraction
2. To gain further understanding and wisdom of the sexual mysteries
3. To increase the membership of the O.T.O.
4. To obtain wealth and the leisure to explore the sexual mysteries more deeply
5. To create invisible bodyguards/warriors so you can perform sex magick without interruption
6. To achieve the Knowledge and Conversation of the Holy Guardian Angel
7. To devote yourself to the gods, particularly Nuit-Babalon-Baphomet, and to gain spiritual attainment
8. To obtain knowledge and insight into Nature and the laws of nature
9. To found an abbey of Thelema
10. To establish the kingdom of Ra Hoor Khuit

Elsewhere, in an unpublished document, Crowley lists seven operations under the rule of the seven planets of the ancients; this list is, in essence, identical to Randolph's list of seven operations above. This is one of the few points that indicate a real connection between Randolph's system and Crowley's. Crowley may, in fact, have received Randolph's system virtually verbatim from Reuss and Kellner, with the addition of the idea of the Eucharist from Reuss with his neo-Gnostic interests. To this, Crowley added his own wonderful Qabalistic creativity, and the praeter-human intelligences with whom he had developed relations.

Crowley saw sex magick as work appropriate to adepts—very advanced magicians—and believed that much preparatory work in ritual and yoga was prerequisite to becoming a sex magician. In the A∴A∴, a huge number of practices are engaged in before the idea of sex magick even comes up. We will explore a number of these preparatory practices in the next few pages.

The G∴B∴G∴

In 1931, a small advertisement appeared in the *Occult Digest* that read simply:

> A shortcut to initiation
> The Choronzon Club

An address was provided for interested parties. This marked the beginning of the G∴B∴G∴, a sex-magick group founded by C. F. Russell, one of Aleister Crowley's former students. The G∴B∴G∴ was active for less than a decade, and probably would have been lost to history except for the efforts of Louis Culling. An early member of the G∴B∴G∴, Culling published all of the order's teachings several decades later. It is rumored that the current Frater Superior of O.T.O. once said, "I wouldn't want to have his karma," when speaking of Louis Culling. And it is true that Culling certainly broke the seal on something very secret and special. He was the first person to publish sex-magical teachings based on the work of Aleister Crowley. Today, this may seem inconsequential, since many of Crowley's most secret writings have seen print again and again. But when Culling broke the oath of secrecy, it was very significant.

The sex magick of the G∴B∴G∴ differed in several respects from Crowley's techniques, however. They modified Crowley's work to suit their own needs. There was no element of masturbation in G∴B∴G∴, or any teachings regarding homosexuality. The work was divided into three degrees—Alphaism, Dianism, and Qodosh—and these degrees have no clear relation to any other degrees in any other system.

ALPHAISM

Alphaism is the name given to "magical chastity" in the G∴B∴G∴. When Culling writes of chastity, he does not refer to celibacy at all, but rather to a very specific attitude toward sexuality that changes your relationship with sex into something magical. There are several ways of approaching magical chastity; the definition provided by Culling and G∴B∴G∴ teachings is really only one. We will discuss some of the other ways of being magically chaste elsewhere.

For the G∴B∴G∴, you practice magical chastity simply by forcing yourself to have no sexual thoughts, feelings, or fantasies except in relation to sex magick or when specifically engaged in sex magick. In other words, you don't think or act sexually unless you are with your partner directly performing an act of sex magick. According to Culling, this type of magical chastity is necessary to approach the next two degrees properly. Before attempting this practice of magical chastity, magick students must learn a number of magical exercises, including dream recall, focusing techniques, and some ritual activities. By training your mind to move along specific pathways under the direction of your will, you learn to control your mind, and hence to avoid thinking about sex outside of your magical operations. The specific practice of Alphaism is not conducted by itself, however, but as part of the work of the next two degrees.

DIANISM

Dianism is the first level of sexual practice in the G∴B∴G∴. Before engaging in the practices of Dianism, you are expected to be an observer of Alphaism. The specific practice of Dianism is basically just sexual intercourse without orgasm. It is similar to any neo-Tantric or *karezza* activity except for a few points. In Dianism, the orgasmic reflex is held in and redirected into aspiration toward the Holy Guardian Angel, the higher divine genius or personal dæmon. We will discuss the Holy Guardian Angel at length in the next few chapters.[30] Sexual stimulation in the practice of Dianism can be active, arduous, and passionate, but all this energy must be directed toward the Holy Guardian Angel, and orgasm must be strictly prevented—at least for males. Females may have orgasms if they want in this system. This is one of several points of sexism within the system. After some practice, the fires of aspiration ease the sexual tension, and you can direct all your energies toward your magical goal. In Dianism, you regard your partner as a god or goddess, a physical manifestation of your Holy Guardian Angel. You avoid thinking of the Earthly personality of your partner at all, making him or her just the anonymous avatar of a divine lover.

The purpose of these activities is to lead you into a deep trance state, called the "borderland" in the terminology of the G∴B∴G∴. In every essential, this "borderland" is equivalent to the Sleep of Siloam that we will discuss later. This state can produce sublime spiritual visions and a greater connection with the Holy Guardian Angel. According to Culling, it may take one or two hours of lovemaking to attain this borderland state, though it may also take less time. Thirty minutes is the minimum, practically speaking.

Like Alphaism, Dianism is not necessarily considered an end in itself, but leads to the practices of the third degree. The only end sought in Dianism is a deep and profound connection with the Holy Guardian Angel.

QODOSH

Qodosh is essentially the same as Dianism in practice, except that, at the end of an extremely prolonged period of lovemaking, you release your orgasm. The point of the Dianism is to connect you more fully with the Holy Guardian Angel and hence the True Will, and also to develop a strong control of the orgasm reflex. Once these two points are established, Qodosh becomes the main magical technology of the G∴B∴G∴.

Just as in Crowley's system, the charged sexual fluids are considered an elixir or Eucharist, eaten at the end of the rite or placed on a talisman of some sort. Within the G∴B∴G∴, Qodosh was used for a number of purposes:

- To invoke a desired human quality or character trait like wisdom, love, imagination, or beauty. Both participants simply think about the desired quality, then eat the combined sexual fluids.
- To obtain some desired end through a letter by putting the sexual fluids on it, preferably with some sort of seal or sigil smeared on, and then sending the letter to the party involved.

- To attract wealth by putting sexual fluids on money.
- To obtain the Knowledge and Conversation of the Holy
  Guardian Angel. This differs from Dianic practice in that, when
  you eat the fluids, you put the Holy Guardian Angel energy
  directly and materially into your body, thus making a physical
  connection with the energies invoked.
- To increase your skill in divination, intuition, or psychic
  development.

Crowley engaged in most of these practices in his own sex magick, and
C. F. Russell clearly just adapted what he'd learned from his old teacher.
Culling, however, added the following advice to his practitioners:

- Take great joy in the sex.
- Let sex be calm and easy.
- Don't lust after ecstasy. Just let it come, as it will.
- Don't be obsessed with the sensation. Instead, let sensation
  transmute into union with the divine lover.
- Have a peaceful and contented feeling in the sex.
- Allow the sexual desire to remain, but direct the energy toward
  the Holy Guardian Angel.
- Speak no words aloud during the rite. Pre-arrange a nonverbal
  signal to slow down if things get too intense.
- Don't ever think of your human partner, but rather see your
  partner as a vehicle of the divine.

Neo-Taoist and Neo-Tantric Sex Practices

Though very rich in ideas and useful information, these Western systems all lack certain elements. First, while they instruct you to control
orgasm, they provide no clear instructions for how to do this, or for
how or where to direct the sexual energy in your body to avoid or
prolong orgasm. Moreover, they all disregard female orgasm as anything other than a novelty. In fact, all of these Western systems completely fail to address the flow of energy in the body in all but the most
basic terms. Aleister Crowley was certainly aware of the Eastern chakras
and similar energy systems, but provides very little practical instruction
in any of his writings about how to open and channel these inner forces.
Interestingly, it seems from the little I've read about Karl Kellner and
Theodore Reuss that these two men focused a good deal more attention on the chakras in their sexual work than Crowley. Perhaps the

upper-degree secrets of O.T.O. contain a rich storehouse of never-revealed instructions about the flow of sexual energy through the chakras. This information is hard to come by, however.

Luckily, a number of neo-Tantric and neo-Taoist materials have been made public in the last decades that concentrate on these areas. They also provide a number of tools for awakening and directing your natural sexual and spiritual energies, along with a number of instructive ideas on what to do with the energies raised if you are trying not to have an orgasm. There are specific regions of your body that can more naturally store these energies than others, and we will discuss them in the coming chapters.

From the East, we can also gather instruction in sexual technique, particularly how to improve your control over the orgasmic reflex, how to please your lover, and how to work through some of the various dysfunctions from which so many suffer. While I personally prefer the active work of the West, we can gather much gold from the fertile East, giving us a very complete palette of sexual powers.

All three of the Western sex-magick systems we have discussed hold that you must become a magician before you can become a sex magician. Though their specific methods for developing these skills differ, they share the same list of prerequisite abilities:

- The ability to focus, control, and direct your mind
- The ability to enter into a magical state
- The ability to visualize
- The ability to travel on the inner planes in the body of light
- The ability to conduct ritual practices and gestures

There are also several abilities more specifically connected to sexuality that must be developed, but we will discuss them in the next two chapters. The following techniques give you some proficiency in magical training and basic ritual magick.

The Magick Trance

The magical trance state has been called by many names: the light trance, light self-hypnosis, magical consciousness, the altered state, day-dreaming, meditation, introspection. It is, however, simply a state of consciousness in which you limit your attention, relax, and focus on imaginary phenomena. You move into this state naturally when you watch TV or a movie, do housework, make love, drive on the highway, daydream, or meditate.

For sex magick, you don't need to enter a trance formally; it will come upon you naturally. But while you are training, it is a good idea to get used to attaining this state through practice. Once you get used to it, you can enter it virtually at will.

Entering a Magick Trance

1. Find a time and a place where you will not be disturbed for at least a half hour. Sit in a comfortable position and allow yourself to relax. Close your eyes.
2. Take three or four deep breaths and allow your body to relax deeply with each exhalation. Then turn your breathing back to your subconscious.
3. Begin to observe your body's sensations. Begin by focusing on your feet. What sensations do you feel? Are they tense? Allow them to relax. Slowly observe and attempt to relax each part of your body, moving upward. Observe your ankles, your shins, your thighs, your buttocks, your groin, your back, your chest, your shoulders, your neck. Continue until you reach the crown of your head. You may become completely distracted by thoughts while you are doing this. Don't worry. Simply resume where you left off when you remember what you are supposed to be doing. By the time you reach the top of your head, you will have achieved a fairly good degree of inward focus.
4. Begin to focus on the area directly above your head, imagining a globe of bright white light a short distance above you about the size of a grapefruit. This is the light of your super-conscious mind. It is the light of your personal Kether, the Qabalistic Crown. It is the *sahasrara*—the thousand-petaled lotus of yoga. Your visualization of this light need not be perfect; just pretend that you are doing it right.
5. Imagine this light shining down upon your head. As the light touches your head, it begins to fill it with light. As this light further relaxes the top of your head, your forehead, eyes, cheeks, jaw, and the back of your head, mentally say to yourself, "ten."
6. Allow the relaxing light to continue filling you. As it moves down to your neck and throat, relaxing them, say "nine."
7. Allow the relaxing light to continue filling you. As it moves down to your chest and shoulders, relaxing them, say "eight."

8. Allow the relaxing light to continue filling you. As it moves down to your arms, hands, and fingers, relaxing them, say "seven."

9. Allow the relaxing light to continue filling you. As it moves down to your belly and back, relaxing them, say "six."

10. Allow the relaxing light to continue filling you. As it moves down to your groin and buttocks, relaxing them, say "five."

11. Allow the relaxing light to continue filling you. As it moves down to your thighs, relaxing them, say "four."

12. Allow the relaxing light to continue filling you. As it moves down to your knees, relaxing them, say "three."

13. Allow the relaxing light to continue filling you. As it moves down to your shins, relaxing them, say "two."

14. Allow the relaxing light to continue filling you. As it moves down to your feet and toes, relaxing them, say "one."

15. You are now in a good trance state. You may experience odd sensations and should be completely relaxed. If you fall asleep during any part of this, do not worry. Just continue where you left off when you wake up.

      Become acquainted with this state. You may not notice any drastic effects, but just feel relaxed. You've just very slightly changed your perceptual conditions and reduced the usual overwhelming number of signals from your physical body. You will still be aware that you are sitting in a room, but that will not be the center of your focus. Simply observe this for a few minutes.

16. After a few minutes, when you feel comfortable, return to normal waking consciousness. To come out of the trance, simply reverse the process. Gradually become aware of your body, reawakening it. Finally, open your eyes and stand up. You will probably feel very relaxed. Record your experiences in your journal.

      When you shift into trance, you may notice a tingling sensation, warmth, coolness, a sense of lightness, a sense of heaviness, a lack of desire to move, minor twitches in your fingers or toes, a feeling of slipping, or a sense of floating. Just a brief time in this state can be as refreshing as a nap.

The Vitality and Energy of Breath

Your breathing is one of the most important ways that you receive energy from the outside world. *Prana*, after all, means both energy and breath. Although it is true that energy is attached to the oxygen you breathe, when you breathe, you also open yourself up to energy in other mysterious ways. Breath is the key to vitality, yet we often ignore it.

Breathing in Awareness and Energy

1. Sit or lie down somewhere where you won't be disturbed.
2. Enter a magical trance.
3. Observe your breath as it enters your body. Feel the cool sensation as breath passes through your nostrils. Follow the air down through your body as it descends deep into your belly. Fill your lungs completely with each breath. First allow your stomach to fill, then your chest, until finally your shoulders feel as if they are filled with air. Be sure not to fill your lungs so much that it's painful. This should be a pleasant sensation, not a forceful battle.
4. When your lungs are full, begin to exhale. This time, begin at the bottom of your lungs, pushing the air out of your belly. Slowly push all of the air out, working upward until your lungs are completely empty. Again, remember to stop before it becomes painful.
5. Consciously visualize the vitality in the air surrounding you. You can see it as sparkles or as a soothing glow.
6. As you breathe in, feel this vitality enter your body. Don't just feel it in your lungs; let it permeate your whole body. Feel the vitality enter through every pore of your body. Take complete breaths that penetrate down to your belly and up to your shoulders.
7. As you exhale, imagine that the toxins you've accumulated through the day exit through every point of your body. Exhale every ounce of air, completely emptying your lungs.

Repeat this for several minutes. You may become distracted with other thoughts, but when you realize that you've become distracted, simply come back to the exercise. When you decide to stop, notice how you feel. Record your experiences in your journal.

Active Imagination and Visualization

One of the most important skills you need to develop as a magician is the ability to create and sustain images in your mind as realistically as possible. This is the way that all magick is conducted. You don't have to visualize anything perfectly, but you do need rudimentary visualization skills to conduct any effective magick. These steps are a simple way to develop your inner visualization skills.

Creating Inner Visualizations

1. Sit or lie down somewhere where you won't be disturbed.
2. Enter a magick trance.
3. Notice what you see behind your closed eyes—a fuzzy grayness, dots of light, or perhaps pictures forming. Describe it to yourself consciously. This will spark your subconscious to throw up more and more images.
4. As more images pop into your mind, describe them to yourself and connect with them through your other senses. Imagine how the fleeting images you see might feel or sound or taste or smell. Just let your imagination flow. The images may only last a moment or two. Call them back by imagining that your senses are interacting with them.
5. As the images become more and more tangible, begin holding onto them. Allow scenes to develop. Continue to describe these scenes in as many different sensory terms as possible. Whole "dreamlets" may begin to emerge.
6. Begin to adjust the contents of these dreamlets, adding elements of your own. Keep doing this for as long as you like. Return to normal consciousness whenever you are ready. Record your experiences in your journal.

After a few tries, you will become quite adept at creating inner scenes at will.

Your Body of Light

Much has been made of astral projection by a wide variety of writers. For magical purposes, you need master only a very rudimentary form of astral projection. In fact, all you need is basically an extension of the visualization exercise you just conducted. The experience has been called clairvoyance, traveling in the spirit vision, or the body of light. This is essentially the same technique used by the famous psychic Ingo Swann, one of the developers of remote viewing, as well as by Aleister Crowley and the initiates of the Golden Dawn. This technique empowers you to imagine yourself into a "body of light." It may all seem totally subjective, but pretending is real to all of your consciousness except for your waking mind. Over time, you may become skilled enough to lose all sense of your body and become completely involved in your visions.

Accessing Your Body of Light

1. Sit or lie down somewhere where you won't be disturbed.
2. Enter a magical trance.
3. Imagine the focal point of your consciousness shrinking, so that your whole consciousness is in the center of your being. You may associate this center at your belly, your heart, or in your forehead—whichever is easiest for you to imagine. Don't worry if it seems as if you're just pretending.
4. Imagine a shape resembling your body made out of light and floating a few feet above you. Allow this shape to become just like you—an image of yourself made of light.
5. Move your point of consciousness into the body of light.
6. Associate yourself with this new body, looking around the room from this new perspective. See your body sitting or lying immobile a few feet away from you. Look down at your body of light; see your hands and feet made out of light particles.
7. Move away from your body and examine the objects in the room around you. Again, this may seem like a mere daydream, but continue pretending.
8. Go out of the room and look around the rest of the building you are in.
9. Go anywhere you wish.
10. When you are ready, return to your body and slowly re-associate, imagining that your body of light re-enters your body. Record your experience in your journal.

The Power of God Names

In various rituals, you are asked to "vibrate" appropriate divine names. This is a simple technique you can master using the following exercise. This creates a powerful magical effect, transforming your speech into magical projection.

Vibrating God Names

1. Imagine the divine name in shimmering white letters descending down into your heart from the globe of white light that crowns you as you inhale.
2. As you exhale, say the name slowly and melodiously, causing a vibration as you imagine the white-light letters going out with your breath. As you intone the name, imagine that a thousand voices bellow forth the word across the heavens.
3. If you are using Hebrew formulae, imagine the Hebrew letters themselves if you can. The same goes for Greek and other scripts. Record your experiences in your journal.

The Assumption of God Forms

You won't need this skill until later, but since it often accompanies the vibration of god names in magical instructions, I give it here. The assumption of god forms is simply a way of connecting astrally with the forms of the gods so that you can represent them in various ceremonial contexts. While this technique is basically just a form of active imagination, it can have a powerful magical and psychological effect on consciousness. It can be used effectively with any pantheon of gods—Greek, Roman, Egyptian, Celtic, or Hindu.

You can also use a modification of this simple technique to connect directly with the archetypal energies of the gods to develop new abilities or personality traits in yourself. Combined with the sexual techniques given later in this book, this can have an incredible transformative power.

Before you begin, familiarize yourself with the characteristics and common physical images of the god with whom you choose to work. The Internet can be an excellent resource for this type of research. Know the form of your god very well, so that you can imagine it as vividly as possible. Crowley suggests that you paint or draw the god so that you are connected with it as deeply as possible.

Assuming the God Form

1. In a magical trance, and probably after conducting some preliminary rituals, begin to visualize the distinctive form of the god you have chosen. See this form glowing intensely with an appropriately colored energy.
2. Move into the same position as the god. Imitate the way you see the god standing, sitting, or moving.
3. Imagine the form of the god moving into and encompassing your form.
4. See and feel yourself and the god integrating into one form. Allow yourself to grow in stature to fill up the universe in the form of this god. Experience the universe as this god would. Become the god as much as possible.
5. Conduct whatever magick you choose in the form of this god.
6. When you are finished with your ritual, separate from the god and thank it for sharing its being with you. Record your experiences in your journal.

The Elements and the Planets

Most practical magical work is categorized as either elemental or planetary. Even if your work takes you beyond these basic principles, they still form the core of most modern magical systems. Most people are at least vaguely familiar with the four elements—fire, air, water, and earth—since they have been a part of the Western magical tradition for thousands of years. The basic qualities of the elements are:

Fire	warmness and dryness, and the quality of expansion
Water	coldness and wetness, and the quality of contraction or shrinking
Air	warmness and moistness, and the quality of lightness
Earth	coldness and dryness, and the quality of heaviness

These ideas and the subtle forces behind them can be used to create dramatic changes in yourself and the world. Fire energizes, water calms, air inspires, and earth manifests. Table 1 gives a few practical ways to direct these four elements in your magick.

Table 1. Magical Purposes of the Four Elements

Fire	inspiring success, creating passion, obtaining and improving sex, creating sexual love, enhancing creativity, developing strength, strengthening will
Water	creating friendship, attracting and understanding love, increasing tranquility, assisting with emotional and spiritual healing, calming or changing emotions, getting needed rest, improving understanding
Air	increasing education, improving memory, enhancing intellect, learning and teaching, improving communication, encouraging travel, inspiring writing, developing new theories, organizing your things
Earth	attracting money, obtaining jobs, getting promotions, improving investments, building your physical health, increasing business, building and enhancing your physical body, constructing buildings and plans, improving physical appearance, understanding and making peace with materialism

The forces of the seven ancient planets are also an important part of practical magick. Of course, these forces do not come directly from the planets themselves, but are rather archetypal ideas attached conceptually to the poetic concepts of the planets.

Moon	imagination, instinct, subconscious, emotion
Mercury	reason, communication, logic, knowledge
Venus	love, passion, aesthetics, nurture
Sun	beauty, harmony, balance, wholeness
Mars	justice, strength, force, violence
Jupiter	generosity, abundance, leadership, vision
Saturn	structure, limitation, seriousness, responsibility

Table 2 gives a few practical ways you can direct the planetary energies to your magical purposes.

When conducting practical magick with these planetary and elemental energies, you create connections with them through objects and visualizations that are congruent with the energies. One of the

Table 2. Magical Purposes of the Seven Planets

Moon	increasing imagination, improving instinct, connecting with the subconscious, altering and developing emotion, connecting with the astral world, developing clairvoyance, enhancing dreams, getting sound sleep, working with the sea
Mercury	developing reason, improving communication, becoming more logical, gaining hidden knowledge, success in examinations and tests, safety and speed in travel, success in business, improving writing, getting into and succeeding in school, learning science, medicine, or mathematics, developing the mind, self-improvement in general, understanding statistics or calculations or systems
Venus	gaining love, creating desire, improving and developing aesthetics, becoming more nurturing, enhancing beauty, increasing pleasure, appreciating and creating art, creating luxury, enhancing femininity
Sun	creating harmony, improving balance, establishing and understanding wholeness, developing friendships, improving health and vitality, regaining youth and beauty, finding peace, experiencing illumination, obtaining windfalls of money, divine power
Mars	bringing justice to a situation, developing strength and passion, applying force, understanding and directing violent urges, enhancing energy, creating or stopping war or warlike thoughts, using aggression, developing courage, winning in competitions, improving in athletics, enhancing masculinity
Jupiter	increasing generosity, creating and understanding abundance, developing leadership skills, becoming a visionary thinker, receiving favors, acquiring influence and prestige, acquiring wealth, solving legal issues, getting good luck, personal expansion
Saturn	understanding and creating structures, overcoming or creating limitations, developing responsibility, becoming more serious, understanding reincarnation, understanding death, receiving inheritances, extending life

best places to find such correspondences is in Aleister Crowley's book 777. You can choose appropriate incense, colors, geometric shapes, gemstones, plants, gods, and many other things to create an environment that instantly calls to mind the energies of these concepts.

One of the easiest ways to create an appropriate atmosphere for working with these energies is with color. The effect of color on consciousness is very powerful. It is often enough by itself to ensure connection with the proper mood. Table 3 gives the traditional color correspondences.

When you build up these colors powerfully in your imagination, you form a wonderfully conducive atmosphere for your magick. You can also use colored cloths and candles in your work area to augment your imagination and empower your rites.

Table 3. Elemental and Planetary Color Correspondences

Fire	red or red-orange
Water	blue or blue-green
Air	yellow or blue
Earth	green, black, or brown
Saturn	black or indigo
Jupiter	blue or violet
Mars	red
Sun	yellow or gold
Venus	green
Mercury	orange or mixed colors
Moon	violet, blue, or silver

Little Rituals for Magical Development

The next six exercises give you the basics of ritual magick. They should probably accompany most of your practical work in some form. They can be conducted very informally without losing their effectiveness.

Before almost any important magical work, purify yourself to clear away the negative energies of the day's events and bring your consciousness into focus on the magick you are about to do.

Purifying Your Energy

1. Enter a magical trance.
2. Take a small bowl of water in your hand, or immerse yourself in a bath.
3. Sprinkle some of the water on yourself, letting go of all things that don't relate to the work, saying to yourself: "I cleanse myself, so that I may purify myself, so that I may accomplish my work," or something similar. You can also specifically mention the work you are about to do. Or you can use the traditional Latin: *Asperges me, Dominus, hyssopo, et mundabor; lavabis me, et super nivem dealbabor*, or Crowley's suggested: ". . . pure will, unassuaged of purpose, delivered from the lust of result, is every way perfect."
4. Visualize and feel the water sucking away all negativity.

This simple technique becomes more and more powerful as you use it. Repetition builds an accumulation of power. The same holds true for ritual consecration. Purification rids you of unrelated or negative thoughts; consecration dedicates you to the work at hand. As purification is to water, consecration is to fire.

Consecrating the Work

1. After purifying yourself, take some incense in hand.
2. Place your body and face into the smoke of the incense. Smell it and feel the warm tickle of it filling you, saying something like: "I consecrate myself to this work, and this work alone, that it may be accomplished with the power of the great animating consciousness of the universe." Or you can use the Latin: *Accendat in nobis Dominus ignem sui amoris et flammam aeternae caritatis,* or

Crowley's, "I am uplifted in thine heart; and the kisses of the stars rain hard upon thy body."

3. Feel and visualize the light from your crown filling your whole body as you speak.

Magical weapons and tools are usually consecrated in a similar manner. In sex magick, you can consecrate your work by rubbing sexual fluids on objects rather than simply using incense smoke. Of course, you can also do this as part of your own consecration— but that would put the cart before the horse in most cases.

Even if you conduct your magick fairly informally, you should separate it from the rest of your life. The simplest way to do this is by creating a magical circle. You can do this before, after, or sometimes instead of purification and consecration.

Casting a Magical Circle

1. Get into a magick trance.
2. Imagine the globe of light above your head entering your body and moving down your arm. Imagine the light flowing into your shoulders and down your arm into your outstretched fingers. Develop a very strong sense of this light powerfully flowing into you from above.
3. Go to the east of your work area. Point your hand down at the ground, imagining the light coursing from above, through your arm, and projecting down to the ground.
4. Slowly walk the perimeter of the room clockwise, tracing a glowing line of energy on the floor as you go.
5. When you get back to the east, finish the circle and move to its center—the center of the room.
6. Allow the light to continue flowing into you. Imagine that it begins to accumulate in your heart. Visualize it as a bright ball. Let it continue growing and expanding until it expands past your body.
7. Set this light spinning counter-clockwise. As it continues to grow, imagine that the turning light sweeps away all outside energies.
8. Continue this visualization until the globe of light fills the whole circumference of your circle, reaching above your head and

below the earth to completely surround you with a globe of light.

All extraneous energies have now been swept out of your working area. You can also go through this procedure in your mind, in your body of light, once you're familiar with it, imagining the whole circle and sphere into existence without ruining any romantic mood you are trying to set up with your sex partner.

The following rituals are a bit more elaborate, but they are useful in work pertaining to the elements and the planets. We will expand on these rituals with visualizations and additional information later, but for now, just familiarize yourself with their structure.

You can use the next ritual in addition to or instead of circle-casting. Many people use invoking pentagrams at the start of their rituals and banishing pentagrams at the conclusion. Others simply begin and end with the banishing pentagrams.

Lesser Ritual of the Pentagram

1. Facing east, touch your forehead and say, "Ateh."
2. Touch your breast and say, "Malkuth."
3. Touch your right shoulder and say, "ve-Geburah."
4. Touch the left shoulder and say, "ve-Gedulah."
5. Clasp your hands on your breast and say, "le-Olahm, Amen."
6. Go to the east edge of your magick circle, and trace a large invoking or banishing earth pentagram with your outstretched finger (see figure 3). Vibrate the name "IHVH."

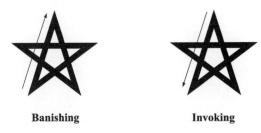

Banishing   **Invoking**

Figure 3. Earth pentagrams

7. Turn to the south and trace a large invoking or banishing earth pentagram. Vibrate the name "ADNI."

8. Turn to the west and trace a large invoking or banishing earth pentagram. Vibrate the name "AHIH."
9. Turn to the north and trace a large invoking or banishing earth pentagram. Vibrate the name "AGLA" (Ye-ho-wau, Adonai, Eheieh, Agla).
10. Extend your arms at your sides like a cross and say: "Before me Raphael, behind me Gabriel, On my right hand, Michael, On my left hand, Auriel, For about me flames the Pentagram, and in the Column stands the six-rayed Star."
11. Repeat steps one through five.

The easiest way to invoke the energies of the planets and the elements is with the greater rituals of the hexagram and the pentagram inherited from the Hermetic Order of the Golden Dawn. In these rituals, each point on the pentagram and the hexagram are assigned to particular energies—pentagrams to invoke and banish elemental energies, and hexagrams to invoke and banish the energies of the planets. These two rituals may seem confusing at first glance, but they are really very simple (see figure 4).

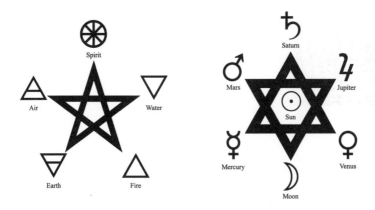

Figure 4. Elemental pentagram and planetary hexagram

Greater Ritual of the Pentagram

Before tracing the elemental pentagrams, invoke the ruling element of spirit, using the pentagrams, symbols, and divine names shown in figure 5. When invoking water or earth, use the passive-spirit pentagram. When invoking fire or air, use the active-spirit pentagram. Then trace the elemental pentagrams representing the element you wish to invoke,

adding the appropriate symbols in the middle and vibrating the appropriate divine names (see figure 6).

In order to invoke any element, simply trace the appropriate pentagram in the four quarters, along with the symbol at the center, and
vibrate the appropriate divine name. At the end of your ritual, banish
the energies, reversing the energy (see figure 7). Then use the banishing spirit pentagrams shown in figure 8.

Greater Ritual of the Hexagram

This ritual is easily performed. Simply trace the appropriate hexagram
in the four quarters, vibrating "Ararita" and the appropriate god name.
The unicursal hexagrams of the planets, with their divine names, are
given in figure 9.

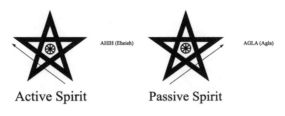

Figure 5. Invoking spirit pentagrams

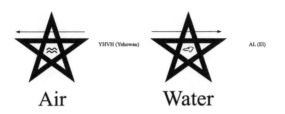

Figure 6. Invoking elemental pentagrams

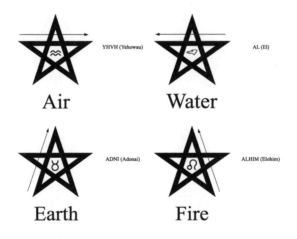

Figure 7. Banishing pentagrams

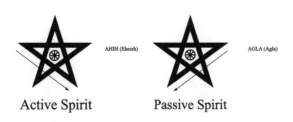

Figure 8. Banishing spirit pentagrams

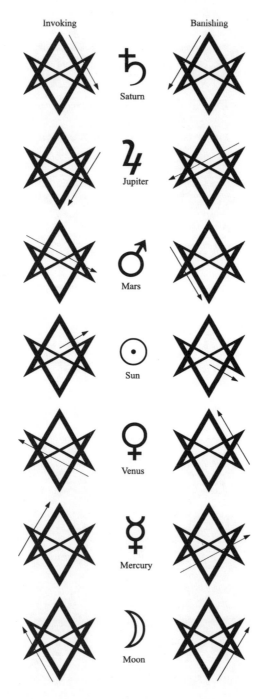

Figure 9. Unicursal hexagrams of the planets

CHAPTER 3

Sexual Metaphysics

Every man and every woman is a star.

—*Liber AL vel Legis, I, 3*

This chapter is a brief guide to the spiritual connections of gender and biology to human sexuality. Before beginning, however, we'll go over a few basic terms of sex magick that will reoccur through the remainder of the book. Actually, a number of these terms have already come up, but I want to discuss them explicitly before we go any further.

Magical Chastity

Chastity in general is a behavior, or lack of behavior, that creates and preserves purity. In a magical context, however, this does not necessarily correspond to sexual abstinence. We have already discussed this term briefly in the work of the G∴B∴G∴, but there are several related ideas that contribute to the whole of the idea of magical chastity.

The first and most obvious type of chaste behavior is simply to abstain from sex. I did this more or less effectively for a brief time in my late teens, and it did have some useful cumulative effects. By avoiding sex, I found I could connect much more easily with visionary states and remember my dreams more consistently. Although this is a subjective observation, I do think there is a certain amount of validity to it. And I think it is especially true for someone just starting out on the magical path. Having a little extra energy can't hurt. But just holding onto your sexual desire is not very helpful. How much fun can it be to be a sexual sorcerer without sex?

Moving your sexual energy around in your body and transforming it into other kinds of energy is the second type of magical chastity. It is chastity with the aid of technique. In this form of chastity, you can even have sexual intercourse if you refrain from genital orgasm, instead moving the energy up into your body and transforming it into magical and spiritual power. This form of chastity can be called "energetic chastity." Through it, you build rather than expend your energy. You find this sort of chastity in Tantric and Taoist practices, and in the Dianism degree of the G∴B∴G∴.

A third type of magical chastity, described by Louis Culling, requires that you limit your thought about and conduct of sex to a magical context. This form of magical chastity is recommended by both Crowley and Randolph, to greater or lesser degrees. "If he is however, under the influence of carnal passion [when ejaculating], of bestial instinct, the man is suicide, lost demoralized."[31] Crowley also had another concept in mind when he used the term chastity, and we will discuss that in a moment.

This third form of magical chastity, in which you only engage in sex or think about it in a magical context, is very important. In many ways, this simply makes good practical sense, in terms of metaphysical hygiene. If you are going to devote sexual energy to religious and magical practices, why have sex that is not directed in this way? That would be like taking communion in a Catholic church, but also keeping a box of communion wafers by the couch to snack on while watching TV.

If sex is going to be a holy act, why not always make it an act of holiness? I know that many readers already consider sexuality in this way more or less. But let's bring this concept fully into your consciousness. How often has sex or masturbation served merely to scratch an itch? This is not to say that you always have to have some magical purpose in mind when having sex, but rather simply that it should probably always be regarded as a magical sacrament. As I've been preparing this manuscript, a number of people have expressed to me that they would not want someone to be "doing sex magick" without them knowing about it. Well, it seems to me that, if you are a magician in the true sense of the word, then every sex act is going to be a magical act, because it is an expression of your love and your will. This is the essence of magick.

Crowley propounded a fourth type of magical chastity that simply meant doing only those things that are in harmony with the True Will. This is, in many ways, the most important aspect of magical chastity. Sex is only a secondary consideration in Crowley's definition of chastity. His main point is that all acts must be in accord with the True Will. Thus any action you take that goes against your True Will is unchaste.

Crowley encourages practitioners to have sex as often as possible, with any willing partners that appeal to you. He does, however, insist that your sex acts be in accordance with your True Will. You should, therefore, explore only those sexual acts that will not swerve you from your true course in life. This, of course, is a highly subjective matter, and one that you will have to approach through your own conscience and wisdom, and your own understanding of your True Will.

The Holy Guardian Angel–the Divine Genius or Daimon

The Holy Guardian Angel is an archetype—a fundamental concept that will, nonetheless, be different for different people. Plato, in his *Republic* defines the essence of the Holy Guardian Angel in beautiful allegorical terms. We each have a purpose for incarnating—a True Will, something we desire to express or do in the physical world. We are each a functional unit of divine consciousness, and we are here on this material plane to express some particular aspect of divinity. Your soul chooses a daimon, a genius, an angel, a divine guide who best represents this True Will. This angel is your guide through the challenges inherent in life. Without this guide, you would be lost. As your soul readies itself for incarnation, it must drink from the waters of forgetfulness that lie between the realm of souls and the realm of the living. When you are born, you completely forget your destiny—your task. Your daimon reminds you of it and steers you toward your destiny.

The daimon, or Holy Guardian Angel, is your connection with the ultimate consciousness of which you are an expression. You lose the sense of your divinity through your contact with the physical world. You "drink from the waters of forgetfulness" through every interaction that separates you from the things that surround you. Mother refuses you milk, and you forget that you are one with the mother. You burn your fingers on the stove and you forget that you are one with fire and one with the stove. The perceptual framework of material existence quickly robs you of your inherent cosmic nature.

Your Holy Guardian Angel is a unit of consciousness that is above material existence, whose job it is to reawaken your divinity. But it is more than this. The Holy Guardian Angel is all of your spiritual experience, because ultimately, it is your true unconscious self. As all spiritual experience is the unfolding of your self to yourself, your Holy Guardian Angel is both your first and your ultimate spiritual experience.

There is a tradition in the magical worldview that the daimon is a "male" concept and the soul a "female" concept. This is an unnecessary distinction, since these concepts really transcend the common view of physical gender. Just as there is polarity in everything, there is an aspect of the soul that is male. Likewise, in Greek Gnosticism, the feminine counterpart of the daimon is *Ennoia*, which literally means insight. The Holy Guardian Angel is often active, positive, creative, expressive, and instructive, but this does not necessarily mean "male." It merely means that it is those things. Though the Holy Guardian Angel may inspire us, it also passively awaits the activity of the soul, whose work creates the possibility of connection and illumination.

The Magical Child or Bud Will

There is a tradition among Jewish sexual adepts of the Kabbalah that conjugal union is a divine creative act that disturbs the energies of the universe. This creative act, if abused, can cause all sorts of problems, such as attacks by succubae and other unholy creatures. Masturbation is particularly abhorred because it attracts astral larvae to the resulting sexual energies and fluids that are not engaged in the act of procreation. For this reason, Jewish adepts insist that sex acts must be preceded by sincere prayer, and only used with the purpose and intention of procreation.

There is a corollary belief that whatever is in the mind of a man engaged in sex at the moment of orgasm will effect the life of the child produced. If the man is thinking lustful thoughts about his wife and the pleasure of her vagina, he will produce a girl child. If, on the other hand, he focuses his thoughts on creating a son, noble and virtuous, then he will indeed create a son. This is, of course, a completely sexist and rather sad idea in and of itself, but it does have an interesting metaphysical connotation. It is this idea that spawned Crowley's infamous phrase: "A male child of perfect innocence and high intelligence is the most satisfactory and suitable victim."[32]

Instead of creating a physical child of either gender in your sex magick (unless that is your goal!), you can use your creative will to manifest a desired goal. You sacrifice a potential "wonderful son," and take and eat the sexual fluids, creating a Eucharist, a god-eating sacrifice in an almost Christian sense. You create a "magical child" that is the divine incarnation of your will. If you then eat the sex fluids, you reabsorb that divinity into yourself.

The magical child or bud will is the energetic offspring of your magical will, usually considered to be present in the sexual fluids produced by your rite. According to some accounts, Theodore Reuss generally only consumed a symbolic amount of the elixir—a drop or two, often mixed with brandy. Crowley, on the other hand, eagerly consumed all of it, considering it analogous to the communion of the Roman Catholic Mass. One lost drop was considered a tragedy and a sacrilege.

The Sleep of Siloam

H. P. Blavatsky claimed that the Sleep of Siloam was "used by one of the highest schools of initiates in Asia Minor, Syria, and upper Egypt for one of the processes of initiation. While the candidate was plunged in deep sleep, his spiritual ego was enabled to confabulate with the gods, descend into Hades, or perform works of divinely spiritual character."[33] In sex magick, this generally means a trance created through the sex act, in which the magician enters a highly altered state to conduct visionary magical work or to experience mystical phenomena. It is a sleep of lucidity in which the magician is freed through orgasm or extended sexual exertion from the usual limits of normal consciousness.

In *De Arte Magica*, Crowley describes an extended operation called "Eroto-Comatose Lucidity," in which, "he is attended by one or more chosen and experienced attendants whose duty is (a) to exhaust him sexually by every known means (b) to rouse him sexually by every known means. Every device and artifice of the courtesan is to be employed, and every stimulant known to the physician."[34] It is questionable, however, whether this much effort is really required to get into this state. Elsewhere, Crowley writes, "...but on him that is bodily pure the Lord bestoweth a Solar or Lucid Sleep, wherein move Images of pure Light fashioned by the True Will. And this is called by the Qabalists the sleep of Shiloam..."[35] Thus, if you fulfill yourself fully (i.e., experience orgasmic release), you enter a lucid sleep. You can follow this with gentle sexual arousals to remain at the edge of consciousness and commune with the divine. Or you can just fly free. Randolph also alludes briefly to this phenomenon, calling it "Sialam exaltations."

I should also mention in passing that the Pool of Siloam was a body of water in Jerusalem where Jesus restored sight to a blind man. The metaphysical implication here is obviously that the sight restored to this man was the lucid spiritual vision. The tarot card The Hanged Man is often associated with both water and the Sleep of Siloam. Crowley's version of this card represents a man floating on water; Blavatsky's text describes the bed upon which the adept is plunged into sleep as having the shape of a cross, just like the Hanged Man.

The Magical Link

Two separate but related ideas make up the concept of the magical link in sex magick—and really in all magick. First and foremost, the link is a connection between you and the target of your magick. In its most basic sense, this is usually hair, blood, or some personal item as in the formulae of medieval black magick. This connection has a metaphysical dimension, however, as a pathway of causal connection between you and your target. And this brings us to the second half of the idea of a magical link: There has to be a causal link between you and your magical target.

Suppose that you want Justin Timberlake or Orlando Bloom to fall in love with you. You've even gone so far as to obtain an old Evian bottle that contains his backwashed saliva. There is still no hope of making him fall in love with you if you do not have some kind of causal link. You must know people in common, for instance, or be going to the same party. With no connection point between the two of you, there is little hope of reaching him, even with the most profound acts of sorcery. And even if you do have some sort of connection, you may not have the magnetic pull to attract a Justin Timberlake, because so many people are sending him this sort of energy. The correct force, in the correct amount, directed in the correct way, toward the correct target. This is the essence of the magical link.

In a sense, the sexual fluids you place on a talisman are also a magical link, because they physically link your essence with your intent. Applying the fluids to a talisman creates a link between your expressed desire and the magical will applied through the sex act. However, without the first half of the equation in place, the second half becomes rather dubious.

The Great Work

This term is used in different ways by different authors, and sometimes even in different ways by the same author. It is used to describe personal illumination or development through some sort of alchemical or magical working, and sometimes refers to the illumination and liberation of the world as a whole. It is also used simply to indicate some smaller yet personally important work, such as a magical or sex-magical operation, or even the writing of a book or the creation of a painting. In this book, the phrase will only be used in its most general sense, as a metaphor for personal evolution.

The Great Rite

The Great Rite is the third degree operation of Gardnerian witchcraft. It is a sex-magical rite in which the two participants invoke the powers of a god and goddess and unite sexually to express the connection of the two god forms, experiencing ecstatic union with both. The Great Rite is sometimes acted out symbolically, without sex, by simply placing the blade of the witch's ceremonial dagger (*athame*) into the sacred cup or chalice. This is obviously not at all the same sort of ritual, but many witches seem to derive some sort of benefit from it. There is certainly precedent for this, since Gerald Gardner's original Great Rite is essentially a "witch-ified" rewrite of Crowley's O.T.O. Gnostic Mass, which itself involves a blade and a cup to symbolize the same ideas. True sexual invocation is so immediately powerful and transformative, however, that such a ceremonial imitation seems rather hollow.

The Homunculus

In ancient Qabalistic and alchemical terms, the homunculus is a body without a soul, brought to life through magical methods to act as servant to the wizard. In modern sex-magical terms, it has two separate meanings. Sometimes it is used simply as another name for the bud will or magical child. However, sometimes it refers to a complex working, as in Crowley's novel, *Moonchild,* where a literal attempt is made to incarnate an entity that is elemental or planetary in nature. Such an entity would not have a "soul," but would instead be a physically living elementary. Why anyone would ever want to do this is utterly beyond me.

The True Will

The True Will is simply that which you came into the world to do. It is the job that your daimon, or Holy Guardian Angel, helps you to accomplish. It is the fulfillment of your basic nature. You were born with a certain type of character and at least a vague sense of what you intend to do in this life. You may or may not ever have had any conscious sense of this. And even if you had, it was probably largely squashed by the expectations of parents and your environment.

One of the most important magical accomplishments that you can achieve is to examine yourself thoroughly, both logically and spiritually, to rediscover this inner purpose and then set about fulfilling it. One of the keys to universal knowledge is right recollection of your original self. You must, in a way, become what you were as a small child. You can do this by thinking backward through all of the events of your life, letting them go as you do. You must simply free yourself of their hold on you, and go back.

Gaining the Knowledge and Conversation of your Holy Guardian Angel is, of course, a key component of this. In its most basic sense, your Holy Guardian Angel is your "Unconscious Creature Self."[36] This daimon is sometimes identified as a kind of cosmic phallus—the instrument for expressing the cosmic will, and hence the source of your inner mission. This, however, perpetuates the same sort of cosmic gender politics that create confusion. It is perhaps better to say that it is the active, expressive, creative outpouring of the cosmos as it is reflected in your individuality.

Your True Will always relates to your creativity. You may have incarnated to do any number of things; only you can determine your real destiny. Your True Will always transcends your individual ambition or selfish desires. It is always something that contributes to the whole of the universe, even if it also contributes to you. It may be that your True Will is to become very rich and powerful, but this is only true if your riches and power also contribute to the evolution and economy of the universe as a whole. The next three exercises will start you on your way to realizing your full potential.

Anything is possible for you. I know this about myself more clearly today than ever before in my life. Hopefully, you will come to this delightful truth about yourself as well. Your True Will is waiting for you. It is waiting for you to gain the courage to do what you really want in this life. Nothing stands between you and your dreams but yourself. Your True Will always relates to your natural creativity, although this does not necessarily equate with artistic creativity. It may be that you are creative communicatively, spiritually, mathematically, or in some entrepreneurial way. To discover your True Will, take out your journal and answer the questions in the following exercise.

Discovering Your True Will

1. How does your creativity naturally manifest?
2. What do you wish you could do with your life?
3. What would you do with your life if nothing could stop you from succeeding?
4. What are your most secret fantasies and dreams for your life?
5. Are your fantasies about your life really yours, or were they implanted by your parents, your culture, or your friends?
6. What were you interested in as a child?

The answers to these questions can provide you with a number of clues to your destiny. But much has happened in your life to obscure your original self. You have suffered emotional scars, rejection, and cultural indoctrination, all of which can make your True Will rather murky. Over the next few days, make a list of all of the major events in your life—successes, failures, personal affronts, lectures, training, love affairs, projects, jobs—anything you can think of that has had a significant effect in molding your personality.

Once you have as complete a list as possible, sit in a magical trance and go over these events in your mind, exploring their emotional impact. Then release your emotional attachment to these events. Allow yourself to let go of both positive and negative experiences. This may take several sessions, but when you have completed the task, you will be on your way to understanding your true and original self.

Magical Goals

As you explore your fantasies and your past, start setting some goals for your future. What do you want your life to look like next year, five years from now, fifteen years from now? What do you want to accomplish with your sexual sorcery? Set at least five serious long- and short-term goals for yourself. My book, *The New Hermetics*[37], provides an excellent goal-setting workshop if you would like some structure in this process.

Sexual Metaphysics

Whether you describe the start of the universe as masturbation by the self-created god Atum, as the ancient Egyptians did, or prefer the more modern description of the big bang, it seems clear that the universe exploded into existence in the first orgasmic ecstasy. The universe was infinitely sexual, even at its very beginning. From the atomic particles turning about in desire for one another, to the gravitational whirling of the planets and the stars, the universe is eternally alive with desire.

This desire expresses itself continuously as two equal and opposite forces, drawn to each other by that mysterious power that we artists call love. These polarities are also sometimes associated with good and evil. This duality of nature is a common concept in many religious philosophies, but it can create confusion in the context of sex magick. The metaphysical structure that grounds this book is basically a non-dualistic Gnosticism. Though "evil" may exist to a certain extent in the universe, it is a by-product of the process of existence, not an equal and malevolent force opposing the "good."

POLARITY

It is tempting to view things that you do not like or understand as somehow existing apart from yourself—as an "other" who is out to get you. Accepting the unpleasant as an inherent part of yourself, and as something that must be integrated, requires a much higher level of personal responsibility. While dualism implies the existence of two fundamental and distinct forces, polarity implies a single fundamental entity or force seen from two perspectives. Life contains the polarities of birth and death, but it is still inherently one thing. Male and female exist in polarity, but they are the two parts of one being—the human being—and are not in opposition unless we make them so. Symbolic representations of this polarity appear in many cultures that are not, at heart, dualistic. The yin and the yang of the Tao are just one example of this.

When you externalize positive and negative forces, you begin to extend similar and analogous dualities to your life experiences, and this can become dangerous. Man is active. Woman is passive. Man is positive, woman negative. Although these comparisons can contain a certain amount of valuable insight, they are subject to severe limits. Their validity will depend on your own gender and how you feel about other members of your gender! I've known some women who seem to feel that women are evil, and some who are certain that men are. But there's no realistic way to make these sorts of comparisons. The polarities certainly exist, but they exist in an interwoven blend of polarities that is the tapestry of life itself. There is no way to place one category into a direct and constant relation to any other category.

Your ultimate concept of universal consciousness—God or whatever name you choose for your god—is one singular thing. It transcends all polarities, but, at the same time, contains them. This monad of Godhead, this one thing, is also all things. It contains polarized fundamental concepts no matter how you look at it—singularity and multiplicity, infinite largeness and infinite smallness, infinite knowledge and infinite action, infinite transcendence and infinite immanence. Largeness is always contracting toward nothingness, while smallness is all always expanding toward omnipresence.

Although it contains these qualities, the monad is also beyond these qualities, thus creating another polarity of the perception of Godhead below the transcendent and beyond transcendence.[38] Crowley's *Book of the Law* contains these principles in the form of Nuit, goddess of infinite space, and Hadit, the infinitely small but omnipresent point. In juxtaposition to these, there is Ra Hoor Khuit, the Monad.[39] Ra Hoor Khuit is actually only one half of the concept of Heru-Ra-Ha, the other half of which is Hoor Paar Kraat. Ra Hoor Khuit is the active creative force, while his twin, Hoor-Paar-Kraat, is pure potential as yet unrealized. Hoor-Paar-Kraat is the Babe in the Egg, the infinite possibility of all manifestation, but without direction. This is also The Fool in the tarot. As soon as some direction is chosen, he becomes the active force Ra Hoor Khuit.

This is an important concept in sex magick. At the start of any operation, the magical force you are working with is Hoor Paar Kraat—pure potentiality. As you direct this force into manifestation at the point of orgasm, it becomes Ra Hoor Khuit. Orgasm is an expression of will, whether you explicitly think of it this way or not. This is one of the many reasons why magical chastity forms an important part of your work.

This is one of the key principles of sex magick. Essentially, through the metaphysical power of the sex act, which we will discuss more in a moment, you create a magical child who is an autonomous little god—a little Ra Hoor Khuit—to accomplish your will. The power inherent in sex is Hoor Paar Kraat, and the direction that you send it transforms this potentiality into the force of Ra Hoor Khuit.

These infinite levels of polarity have been recognized in every culture, and are usually given the names of a divine pairing—Shiva and Shakti, Logos and Sophia, etc. The interaction of these polarities manifests the universe. Their activities transform at each level of creation, but the entirety of the universe, from idea to manifestation, is the interplay of these two archetypal ideas. The sources of Logos and Sophia are found in the lofty ideas of word and wisdom, but they are also equally present in the genitals and their function. The word, or Logos, is made manifest through the male orgasm, which initiates the creation of a child. As the fetus begins to form, it is the wisdom, or Sophia, of the uterus and the organs of the woman that form and mold it into a human baby. Yet Logos is present in each woman, and Sophia within each man. These ideas are also present in your own unique psychological makeup as archetypes that inform you of who and what you are.

There is no real division between the two halves of a polarity. Shiva is inherently a part of Shakti, and Shakti inherently a part of Shiva. The polarity occurs in perception, and the mystics often tell us that this perception was created for the expression of love. But perception and love sadly seem to lead rather naturally into less desirable states. Polarity may exist for the expression of love, but its ultimate result is often fear and hate. You fear the loss of your beloved. You don't like what you perceive as different from yourself. As you move farther and farther from the divine to the mundane, the differences between the component elements of the divine consciousness become more and more confused, and the unhappy state of the world of experience comes into existence. When you are consumed with personal doubt and fear, you never see anything but this fear. Ultimately, you *are* Sophia and Logos, Shiva and Shakti, and through the magick of sex you can come closer to glimpsing this transcendent truth.

THE TETRAD

Raphael Patai, in his wonderfully interesting book *The Hebrew Goddess*,[40] points out that, in ancient cosmologies, the sexual polarities are often split into two sets of gods and goddesses—an original mother and father, and their children. We see this in the Qabalistic tetragram YHVH, in which Y is the father, H the mother, V the son, and the final H the daughter (see figure 10).

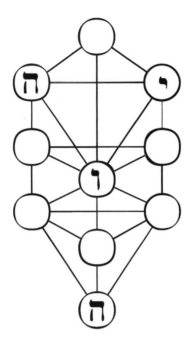

Figure 10. YHVH on the Tree of Life

We also see a divine tetrad in Crowley's metaphysical cosmology—Nuit (the infinite circle), Hadit (the infinitesimal point), Babalon (the all-consuming love), and Chaos (the infinitely creative will). This is not, however, the *tetragrammaton*, which, in Crowley's system, approximates:[41]

Chaos	Y
Babalon	H
Holy Guardian Angel	V
Soul	H

This is just another example of the layers of polarity that exist throughout creation, from our highest archetypal concepts to the most basic atomic structures.

There is an occult tradition that the male is more active in the physical plane, while the female is more passive. There is, of course, a sexual metaphor here. But in this tradition, the female is more active in the astral plane, and the male more passive. This alternating polarity extends up through the various levels of spiritual unfolding, until it

Sephirah	Male	Female
Malkuth	Active	Passive
Yesod	Passive	Active
Hod	Active	Passive
Netzach	Passive	Active
Tiphareth	Active	Passive
Geburah	Passive	Active
Chesed	Active	Passive
Binah	Passive	Active
Chokmah	Active	Passive
Kether	-	-

Table 4. Qabalistic Polarities

Plane	Male	Female
Physical	Active	Passive
Astral	Passive	Active
Causal	Active	Passive
Divine	-	-

Table 5. Polarities in a Four-part Model of Consciousness

finally merges in the inseparable unity of the monad, where the polarity continues to exist only as a potentiality. Tables 4 and 5 illustrate this, although other models contain this same concept as well.

MALE AND FEMALE ARCHETYPES

These concepts of polarity take on the form most relevant to our discussion in the two sexes and their sex organs. It is, therefore, easy to project the essence of your own maleness or femaleness onto many different planes symbolically. In ancient and modern occult literature, the Sun is often compared to man and the Moon and/or the Earth to woman. From a sexual point of view, this does seem to have some validity, or at least a hint of sublime truth impossible to explain in words. Just as the Sun gives forth light and heat that is received by the Moon and the Earth, man gives his sperm to woman. Just as the Moon is cyclical and governs the tides and the times of the month, so woman guides the frequency and quality of sexual connection, controls the selection process of sexual congress, and changes her mood, her body chemistry, and her attitudes over the course of the month. In sex, the man generally takes the more active role, particularly in the pursuit and seduction phase, and the woman is receptive or not—again analogous to the Sun and the Moon (see figure 11). Man is almost always ready for sex; his sunlight is always shining for the opportunity of sexual release. Woman tends to be more changeable—one moment eager for caress, the next introspective and desiring something else.

Many women today find these concepts at least vaguely offensive, and I can see why. They are limited and limiting. Nonetheless, the idea bears meditation, because there appears to be some truth to the matter. The light and heat of the Sun vivify the world. The magnetic and gravitational force of the Moon causes the movement of the ocean tides and the changing weather patterns that make life as we know it possible. In conjunction, they create the rains that nourish the Earth, the dew drops of the infinite.

We tend to be dualistic in our thinking, sorting experiences into categories, seeking patterns. These cosmic metaphors are just another example of this. There is nothing wrong with this tendency, provided that you understand it as metaphor and not some sort of hard and fast rule. I have been pursued by women, and I have also experienced sex in which I was almost completely passive. The metaphor becomes even less reliable in same-sex relationships in which two Suns or two Moons come together. In these loving connections, however, one partner is more the Moon, one more the Sun—or perhaps exchange roles at different phases of the connection.

We all contain both of these archetypes—Sun and Moon, male and female, yin and yang. Ultimately, the Great Work is to unite these oppo-

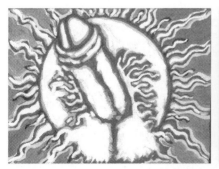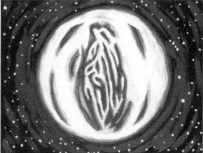

Figure 11. The Sun and the Moon

sites within yourself and transcend them in the realm of pure consciousness. Sexual work of any kind is simply a powerful avenue for exploring yourself dynamically and connecting with these archetypes, within and without, for the purpose of accomplishing this important inner process.

Most ancient religions recognized these archetypes, and many ancient myths are sexual allegories that merit meditation in the hearts of sexual sorcerers. In these traditions, the man—phallus, lingam, or penis—is most often compared to the Sun, and the woman—kteis, yoni, or vagina—is most often compared to the Moon. Many other cosmic symbols play out this relationship between male and female energies as well. The sky and the Earth are often portrayed as in sexual relationship. In Egypt, the sky goddess Nuit has as consort the Earth god Geb. In Greece, the polarity was reversed, and the sky god Uranus consorted with the Earth goddess Gaia. Table 6 summarizes some of the many symbols that have been attached to the male and female energies in different cultures at different times.

Table 6. Symbolic Representations of Male and Female Energies

Male	Sun, sky/Earth, mountain, standing stone, serpent, lion, winged globe, fire, wand or rod, spear, the point, the triangle
Female	Moon, Earth/sky, valley, sea, water, pelican, eagle, egg, cup, flower, the infinite vastness of space, the circle, the triangle

Worshipping the Generative Powers

The worship of generative power is a common practice in India where the Shiva-Lingam is found in many temples and homes, often in conjunction with the yoni of Shakti or Parvati. You can set up a shrine to the generative polarities of the universe in your home, so that you can pay them homage and worship them as you begin your practice of sexual sorcery. Obtain or make suitable images of both polarities, understanding that you are doing this to worship the polarity inherent in the unity of the universe. Your magical goal is to become a worthy channel for your particular polarity, giving due reverence to the opposite polarity and understanding that both are inherent to yourself and the infinite oneness within you. These images can become true talismans of power, radiating the light of the Sun's and Moon's energies into your life from the subtle planes.

You may also worship the Sun and the Moon in the sky, or establish them symbolically in your body, the interior temple of yourself. See the Moon in your generative organs and the Sun in your heart, or imagine the Sun in your generative organs and the Moon in your forehead. Both of these are traditional locations for these polarities in the human body, but you can place them wherever your own instinct imagines them. You are a priest or priestess of these divine powers, and the instruments of your body are perhaps the most fitting ways to worship them. Spend a few minutes each day worshipping the divine polarity in your shrine, in the sky, or in the temple of your body.

The Psychology of Sex Magick

Carl Jung postulated that, within us, we each have a number of archetypal characters that emerge from the collective unconscious. Most important among these are the animus and anima, the masculine and feminine internal archetypes. Jung proposed that every man has an anima, an inner feminine being, while every woman has an animus, an inner masculine being. Modern Jungians have largely modified this view, proposing that both sexes instead possess both internal archetypes. However you approach it, in any relationship you form, these inner archetypal beings play a major role as projections—as idealized images of the opposite sex, as well as parts of your own shadow consciousness that you do not allow to surface.

You most frequently confront these archetypes directly in dreams, where they sometimes take on the guise of your current sexual partner, of idealized or demonized fantasy images. Whenever you encounter an opposite-sex being in dreams, you can be fairly certain that you are dealing with some aspect of animus or anima. Whenever you have a problem with your mate, it is probably a projection of your own inner archetypes. Integration of these archetypal constructs occurs when you withdraw the projections from your partner and begin to deal with these inner forces directly. A number of exercises throughout this book will lead along the path toward this awakening, but let's start at the beginning.

ARCHETYPAL DREAMING AND ACTIVE IMAGINATION

Over the next few weeks, pay special attention to opposite-sex figures in your dreams, whether they are strangers, friends, or lovers. Record your interactions with these dream figures in as much detail as you can recall. Spend a little time analyzing your relations with these dream characters. What messages are they trying to send you? How does this interaction relate to your current romantic life?

Once you have learned a little bit about these archetypal figures from your dreams, conduct the following exercise to make these relations more conscious and productive. Regular conscious interaction with your inner world will help you to evolve very rapidly, both as a human being and as a magician.

Relating to Your Animus/Anima

1. Enter a magick trance. You may also purify, consecrate, and cast a circle, or perform the Lesser Ritual of the Pentagram to get into a magical space.
2. Transfer your awareness to your body of light and travel upward, calling upon your subconscious to return you to the dream realm, where you will be able to interact with the archetypal figures from your dreams.
3. Eventually you will see some sort of scene unfolding before you. Integrate with the scene, whatever it is, and call for your anima or animus.
4. A figure will appear, answering to your call. It may be a familiar figure that you've seen in your dreams, or it may not. It may also change appearance or shape over the course of your interaction. All of this is fine. The way in which it appears to you will communicate information about this archetype. Is it healthy, sad, energetic?
5. Ask the figure to communicate with you, and wait until you feel that it has responded affirmatively. Ask how you can get along with it most beneficially. Ask how it feels about you, your life, your current sex partner. Ask if it has any advice for you. Ask if it will help you accomplish your goals, and work with you in the transformation of your life. If there is anything that confuses you or troubles you about a dream experience with this figure, work it out now.

6. Consider any thoughts that arise to be communication from this figure. The communication may seem to come from a voice outside of your consciousness, or it may seem to be in your own head, in your own voice. No matter how strange the communication appears to be, thank the figure for relating to you.

8. When you feel the conversation is over, say goodbye and return to your body.

9. Perform a banishing Lesser Ritual of the Pentagram, or simply return to normal consciousness.

10. Record your experience in your journal, and seriously consider any information that the archetypal figure related to you.

Your Spiritual Self

This world in which we live is really a fairly toxic place. Everything that we see drives us away from sharing or love. These are viewed as mere abstract fantasies in the world of our experience. All that you see drives you instead toward darkness, separation, and selfishness. Everyday, you take toxins into your body that leave you ill and confused. You are fed ideas electronically and through print that disturb you, fill you with false impressions that lead to the illusory belief that there are differences between all things. You are taught to be ashamed of your body and its desires. You eat food filled with poisons, made in laboratories, made unnatural and unreal. Religion has become a web of treachery and foolishness. All knowledge of the truth and beauty of this universe is given to you freely and naturally by the universe itself, but it is so hard to see beyond the veil of toxicity.

You have been told that you are not the universe. You were told by your parents that you are very small. You cannot conceive of anything except through the medium of yourself. All that you see is just a series of past impressions playing over and over to yourself—each being perceived in the same way it was the last time, in an attempt to cling to something that was never there in the first place.

You are constantly changing. Nothing is ever the same. All that you perceive is really just your own personal chaos, and you cling to past impressions to maintain some weak grasp on the ever-shifting landscape. Modern life is truly the worst kind of madness. Nothing but you and your own experience means anything to you, but you ceaselessly change. You are the only universe you know, and that universe is chaos.

This is not the only way to exist. There are many layers to your consciousness. The outer layer that views the world directly is just the very edge of it. One easy way to peel back these layers of your consciousness is to divide it into discrete parts. For simplicity's sake, we will talk about the four primary layers here, although there are really an infinite number of subtle layers to your mind.

The first layer is, of course, your normal waking consciousness. This is the part with which you are most familiar. The second layer is your subconscious mind, with which you are also probably fairly familiar. This is the part of you that dreams and fantasizes, and drives your habits. The third layer is your super-conscious mind, with which most of us are less familiar. This is essentially the same as your Holy Guardian Angel or dæmon. You access this layer through your subconscious. Many allegories in occult literature describe the marriage of the soul with the spirit, the subconscious with the super-conscious. In the merging of these two, you discover the fourth layer of consciousness—the totality, the great consciousness that forms the whole of the universe. In sexual union, you accomplish a similar merging, and this offers you a similar passage to the divine.

The ocean is a beautiful metaphor for comprehending your relationship with the universe. The ocean is made of billions of molecules of water, but each one is intimately a part of this ocean. You are an individual being, a molecule of consciousness, but you only have function and purpose when conceived as a part of the universe. You can take a cup, dip it into the ocean, and separate a small amount of the water from the ocean. This water is no longer a part of the ocean; it has become instead a glass of water. This is the usual state of the human mind. Humans have lost their sense of connection with the universe, content with being just "glasses of water" separated from the universal ocean. This pronounced sense of individuality has become a prison that scoops each of us out of this ocean of consciousness, and leaves us in our own individual shell or glass.

There is no escape from the universe. It is all-inclusive. Whether you acknowledge it or not, everything that you are is a property of this universe. Your perceptions have merely created the illusion that there is any separation between you and it. This is no way to live. Why choose to be a glass of water, when you can be the ocean? By linking the separate elements of your own consciousness, or linking your consciousness to another through sex, you can dissolve the boundaries in your consciousness and discover the totality.

Consciousness is all there really is, and we are all a part of that one consciousness. Every rock, tree, star, poem, chocolate bar, over-processed junk-food hamburger, annoying liberal, evil dictator, close-minded conservative, children's book, and igloo is part of that one consciousness.

The ego is really a nothing. It is only a point of reference. It is just a means by which you identify yourself. It expands and contracts to suit the caprice of the moment. Sometimes, it concerns itself with your individual well-being; sometimes it includes family or friends. At other times, it grows to envelope a nation, as on the day of the World Trade Center attacks in 2001, when all Americans suddenly felt their egos drawn together in one national consciousness. But the ego is always seeking division. It is Ialdabaoth, the great archon who is the demiurge of the physical world. It is Choronzon, the demon of the abyss of the mind. The ego is present even in exalted states, wherein the master proclaims: "I am one with god. There is no part of me that is not god." At this point, at least in theory, the ego collapses into infinity, but there is still that sense of "I"—the I that is the totality of consciousness itself. The ego itself lacks any defining limits, because it is nothing.

Your conscious mind is just a vessel, a vessel that can contain as little or as much as you allow, depending on your state of mind. Because of your essential connection to everything, your thoughts are very powerful. You may have enabled them to make your world ugly and meaningless, but once you learn to accept the thoughts of your divine genius, your world will be full of your own miracles. Your thoughts do have great power, because you are of the same stuff as the universe. A child of god. Although your thoughts can hide the beauty of the universe or god from you, they cannot destroy or negate it.

Your thoughts can make you healthy, beautiful, and strong. Thoughts are energy. Your body is energy. Your muscles and bones are made of atoms that are just energy. If you direct your mental energy toward your own health and happiness, you can do anything. Your subconscious mind is incredibly good at creating images, both for your benefit and to your detriment. By exploring your soul, your subconscious mind, you gain access to an increasing power over the whole of your consciousness. As you contact your super-conscious mind through your subconscious, through your meditations, fantasies, and magical operations, you gain access to the totality of universal knowledge and power.

The astral, mental, and spiritual worlds are all thought forms. When you construct an image in your mind, it is intensely powerful, because you are powerful. Imagine how powerful the image would be if you truly thought of it as real. Angels, demons, spirits, devils, and gods are all universal thoughts or energies that have been personified by the human ability to turn thought into form. Your thoughts create the physical world you see. It is just energy, without shape. The power of your mind has given it myriad forms. If the world seems a horrible place, look first to yourself for the reason.

The return to universal knowledge is not a loss, but a gain. All that is and was you is taken up into the whole, and you are enriched by all of creation. You remain yourself, as you were, but you become the whole of the universe. The spirit is the divine sea, calm and ordered, from which the chaos of the personal mind flows as a tiny stream.

Imagination is the key to unlock your connection with god. Through it, you can manifest any and all ideas. Eventually, your visualizations take on a life of their own, as the universal mind responds to your gentle prodding. Your soul is your subconscious, the realm of imagination and dreams. Anima and animus, and many other archetypes, dwell in your soul, and it is here that your work begins. By confronting these archetypes, through sexual and emotional interaction with your lover, and directly through visionary work, you begin to unravel the real from the unreal. You awaken your inner world into power and life.

Your spirit is your super-conscious mind. This consciousness will guide your work from the beginning if you let it. The highest archetypes dwell inherently in the lowest archetypes through the process of the unfolding of creation. As animus and anima interact, so do Logos and Sophia, Shiva and Shakti, the divine polarities that create the universe. God is the union of Logos and Sophia, so God manifests in every union. This is true in the connections between beings, and in connections within your own mind and energetic body.

Your Energy Body

All things are connected on an energy level that is neither electrical or physical, and is not confined to time or space. This cosmic energy is consciousness itself, sometimes called *kundalini*, or *chi*, or *orgone*. Call it what you will, it is truly the consciousness of the universe itself that is the fundamental energy. And what drives it? Love. Even your individual physical body, the end of the differentiating process of manifestation, is tuned to the so-called body of God, or the universe at large. Moreover, every part of each human body is connected to all others on an energy level. The simplest and most direct example of this is that, if I take a pin and poke it through my finger, a certain discomfort is felt in all that witness. You may argue that this is "mere sentimentality" or "empathy." But these are just names given to the invisible energy that binds us outside of space and time.

Your body contains many subtle pathways through which all of your energy passes—including electrical, emotional, spiritual, and magical energies. The most important of these passages runs directly through your spine, connecting your whole body electrically and metaphysically at the same time. This passage is the pathway you must travel to find your super-conscious mind and explore your soul. It is also the pathway through which the powers of the universe may be drawn into you. In Indian yoga philosophy, this pathway is known as the *sushumna*. It has also been called many other names throughout the ages—the inner reed, inner flute, the path of kundalini, and the Middle Pillar.

The sex force, your central core, the divine power within you, begins at the base of your spine in and around the area of your generative organs. As you awaken this force within you, it moves more and more actively into your whole body, awakening you to evolutionary experiences of consciousness, spiritual ecstasies, and magical powers. It moves up into your body along the central path of your spine.

When you discover how to manipulate it, this energy operates delicately between your physical and mental sensations, leaning definitely toward the physical. It can be experienced in any part of your body, leading to deliciously pleasant sensations all over. It feels a bit like an internal chill, or a mild orgasmic ripple. The easiest access points for this flow of energy are the top of the head and the base of the spine, or the sex organs. Eastern yogis always begin the energy flow from the lower access point. On the other hand, the Western Middle Pillar exercise and many other rituals draw energy from the crown of the head down. There is no one correct way of accessing this energy. I find it just as satisfying to access it from either direction.

The next two exercises are the most important ones in the book. They deal with the perineum, the small area between your sex organs and your anus. This small muscular region opens and closes the urethra and aids in sexual function, as well as affecting genital function and health in general. The perineum is a critical component of sexuality. A strong perineum increases your sexual sensitivity. It allows women to contract their vaginas, and men to have stronger, more consistent erections. More important, it helps men to resist ejaculation. By mastering this little muscular area, you master sex.

This area is also the base chakra of yoga, the *Mulhadhara* chakra, which means "root support." This chakra is essentially equivalent to the perineum. The goddess Kundalini is said to dwell at the center of this chakra, her tail wrapped three and a half coils around, blocking the entrance of the *sushumna nadi* or central channel of energy, your spinal cord. Your evolutionary sexual power can be released into the rest of your body from this chakra. This power is considered the divine seed of power that Sophia placed at the core of every human to awaken them to their inherent divinity.

"Kegels," (exercises to tone women's perineal muscles) have been a part of the yoga tradition for thousands of years. They are called *mula-bandha*, the root lock. In our context, the mulabhanda is of critical importance because, by focusing on its contraction, you draw your magical energy up through your root or Muladhara chakra into your body, awakening you to greater and greater sexual power and ecstasy. First, however, you must learn to locate and use the muscle.

Finding Your Sexual Energy Gateway

1. Sit or lie down somewhere where you won't be disturbed.
2. Contract and release your perineum muscle a few times. The best way to do this is to imagine that you are trying to hold in urine, but don't squeeze the groin muscle, just the muscle beneath your sex organs. Squeeze that area several times in succession. You may inadvertently squeeze other muscles too—your anus, your groin, your abdominals, your back or shoulders. Just relax, and try to isolate your perineum.
3. Once you are fairly comfortable isolating your perineum, begin to coordinate your breathing with the contractions. Use complete, long, full breaths. As you inhale, contract the muscle, squeezing it as if you are holding in urine. As you exhale, push down on the muscle as if you are forcing out the last drops of urine.
4. After a few repetitions, begin to hold your breath in at your maximum inhalation, and hold your perineum contracted. Then exhale completely, and hold your breath out while pushing down on the muscle for a few seconds. Doing this may produce feelings of sexual arousal. This is a good sign.
5. Record your experiences in your journal.

The next exercise builds directly on the last. You can perform it right after the last one if you wish.

Breathing in Your Sex Energy

1. Sit or lie down in a comfortable place.
2. Take a few deep complete breaths.
3. Continue to breathe deeply, and begin to add the perineum contractions to your breathing. As you breathe in, imagine that your breath is actually coming in through your perineum, or Muladhara chakra, and flowing to your genitals and perhaps up into your belly.
4. As you breathe out, push down on the muscles and imagine that your breath is flowing out through your perineum. Allow this to become as real a sensation as possible. You will know when you have achieved it because you will feel a definite energy in your pelvis. It may be a warmth or a tingling, but it will be unmistakable. It will feel sexual and pleasantly arousing.
5. Relax and enjoy this feeling for a few minutes as you continue to breathe in and out through your perineum region.
6. Record your experiences in your journal.

The Seven Chakras: Gateways of Sex Energy

There are several centers of energy along this inner pathway that attract, contain, and manifest different types of force. Students of this phenomenon disagree as to the number of these centers, their exact location on the anatomy, and the exact function of each. Many books, particularly sexually oriented books, place the first chakra directly in the generative organs themselves, but this is not necessarily accurate. The center that we have already worked with in the perineum is perhaps more accurately the starting point, or perhaps the testicles and ovaries respectively. This is really a matter for personal exploration and discovery. The seven major chakras of yoga philosophy are the most familiar to students, but we will also spend a bit of time with both Chinese and Hermetic models for the energy body.

Most students of occultism are probably familiar with the seven energy centers of Yoga and Tantric philosophy—the chakras. The seven chakras have been adopted into magick and the New Age movement thanks in large part to H. P. Blavatsky's Theosophical Society. They are variously portrayed as mystical globes, whirling energy vortexes, or lotus flowers located along the trunk of the body from the base of the spine to the crown of the head (see figure 12).

The chakras are not physical points, yet they are as real as any other part of your anatomy. They are the seats of your emotional energy and can block or enhance the flow of vitality through you. There is an intimate relationship between the nerve plexuses of your spine and these

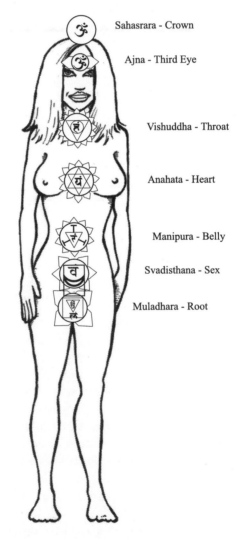

Figure 12. The Hindu chakras

energy centers. You feel your emotions in the regions of each of these chakras. Tension headaches, getting all choked up, love and the pain of love in your heart, butterflies in your stomach, desire in your sexual organs—these emotions all correspond with the locations of the chakras in your body.

Locating Your Seven Chakras

1. We have already discussed the first, or root, chakra, called Muladhara by the yogis. Feel right now in the area between your genitals and anus. Contract the little muscle there for a moment, until you discover that little ripple of sensation. You cannot exercise this muscle too much!

2. The second, or *Svadisthana*, chakra is the sex chakra, located at the base of your sexual organ. Svadisthana means "her special abode." Feel in this area for a moment, until you discover some internal experience in the base of your sex organ. Contract it a little if you wish, until your feel a little ripple of sensation. Feel for a watery, liquid sexual sensation.

3. The belly chakra is called *Manipura*, which means "city of the shining jewel." This chakra is located near your navel. Contract your stomach muscles for a few seconds to locate the sensation, a tingling in your belly. This is sometimes considered a cauldron in which you can store and transform your inner energies.

4. The *Anahata* chakra is the heart chakra, located in your chest. Anahata means, "not struck," which references the mystical inner sounds you sometimes hear in meditation. When you close your ears with your fingers, you can sometimes hear these sounds. When you think about someone you love, you immediately become aware of this chakra.

5. The *Vishuddha*, or throat chakra, is located below the larynx, in the area of the thyroid gland. Vishuddha means, "purified." If you make the sound, "Eeeeeeee," with your teeth not quite together, you can cause a vibration in this chakra.

6. *Ajna,* the third-eye chakra, is located between your eyebrows. Its name means, "command." Intoning the sound, "Mmmmmm," causes a vibration in this chakra.

7. The crown chakra, called *Sahasrara*, is located at the top of your head. Sahasrara translates roughly into "thousand-petaled." This is the entry point for super-consciousness, cosmic power, and

awareness. You have visualized this chakra as a globe of white light above your head in previous exercises, and this is a useful way to approach it.

We all have blocks in varying degrees in some or all of these chakras. In the next chapter, we will actively explore these chakras and their blockages, along with the discoveries of Wilhelm Reich. By exercising and exploring these energetically powerful regions of your body, you will begin to awaken your true sexual power.

The Chinese Energy Body

The Chinese energy body is very similar to the Indian system of chakras in that it contains both energy centers and a central channel. The Chinese approach the cultivation of the sexual energy slightly differently, however, explaining that there are two major meridian lines for energy on the human body. One is called *Tu,* and runs from the perineum up the spine over the top of the head to the roof of the palate. The other is called *Jen,* and runs from the tongue down the front of the body back to the perineum. Energy can be drawn up the spine to the head through the first meridian and then circulated back down to the lower regions along the second. Your tongue must be pressed to the roof of your mouth to achieve this, so you can connect the two meridians in a continuous circuit.

Some Indian practices require this same connection in the palate, and there is certainly a strong connection between the two systems. But while Indian yogis seek to awaken kundalini in a powerful initiatory experience, the Taoists seek to cultivate the movement of energy in the body slowly, through imagination and sensual experience. They focus on the circulation of energy, moving it around the body and storing it in certain areas called *tan tiens.* These energy centers are essentially similar to the chakras, and are often viewed as little alchemical cauldrons within which you can store subtle energies. The main tan tien is in the belly. You cannot store or transform energy in centers higher than the belly until it has been balanced in this lower cauldron. In this, the Chinese and Indian theories are definitely in agreement.

By circulating ching chi (sexual energy) through visualization and physical exercise, you can eventually store this energy and vitalize yourself, transforming it into pure chi, and eventually into the spiritual power that the Taoists call *shen.* Distinctions between chi, shen, prana, kundalini, and the many interpretations of these energy experiences really only create a lot of confusion. They are ultimately one phenomenon. They are all forms and names of the consciousness of love, and that is all that you need to concern yourself with here.

The Taoist technique for circulating these sexual energies is just a part of a much larger program of turning ching into chi, and vitalizing your body. It uses preparatory techniques similar to those we have used earlier in this book. The next exercise is a somewhat simplified version of the full practice.

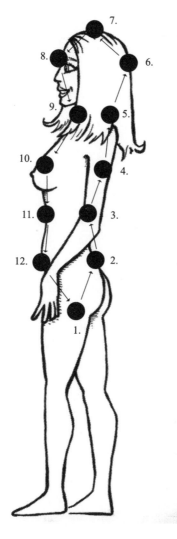

Figure 13. The Chinese Heavenly Circle

The Lesser Heavenly Circle

1. Sit in a comfortable place, close your eyes, press your tongue against your upper palette, and focus inward, entering a magick trance.
2. Begin your sexual-energy breathing, gathering energy in the region of your sex organs. If you want to do this in a properly Taoist way, draw in your stomach as you inhale, and push it out as you exhale (the opposite of natural breathing). But you may breathe in the way that feels most comfortable to you. The important thing is to focus downward toward your Manipura (navel) chakra (the tan tien), while breathing (and contracting your perineum) upward to hold this energy in place. Continue until you feel a build-up of sexual energy.
3. Once you have collected enough energy, but not too much (this is a purely subjective matter; it's up to you), draw the energy back with an intake of breath from your sex organs to the base of your spine (see point 1 in figure 13). This may take more than one breath, but, as you exhale, concentrate on keeping the energy where you want it. On your next inhalation, bring even more energy back to your spine.
4. Bring the energy up to the second point on your spine with your inhalations (see point 2 on figure 13). You will note that these points are at essentially the same places as the chakras.
5. Once you have secured the energy at point 2, continue drawing it up to the other points, until you reach point 7. It is quite likely that the energy will dissipate before you reach point 7. You simply have a few "holes" in your container. Don't worry, the energy is not being wasted; it's patching up the holes! Simply start from the beginning again. Do not try to rush this process, as it will only hinder your development.
6. Once you secure the energy at point 7, move it downward to point 8. To move the energy downward, exhale. It may take more than one exhalation, and the energy may dissipate unexpectedly. If this happens, go back to the beginning. Don't just pull more energy in through your crown. You are trying to make a circle, and cheating won't help you. Push the energy down through each point as you exhale, until you reach point 12 on the figure.

7. When you reach point 12, draw the energy into your lower tan tien (Manipura chakra). The Taoists consider this a very important point, because it is your body's center of balance. Extra energy there will help you with concentration, balance, and martial arts activities.
8. When finished, begin the process over again. You may circulate the energy as much as you feel comfortable in a session.
9. Record your experience in your journal.

Eventually, you will be able to make the whole circle in a single inhalation and exhalation, but don't try this until you're fairly comfortable moving it slowly from point to point. It's easy to fool yourself into believing that you are circulating the energy properly when you are not, so be patient.

The Western Energy Body

The West has many different models for the subtle body, models that have developed at different times in many disparate traditions. Some are planetary or elemental; some relate various forces to certain organs; some relate humors to various actual and imagined bodily fluids; some analyze the body's structures through astrology and the signs of the zodiac.

The model that we will examine most closely is the Qabalistic model of the Tree of Life superimposed on the body, made prominent by the Hermetic Order of the Golden Dawn. This model was recently revived by the writings of Caroline Myss and Golden Dawn student Israel Regardie presented an exercise for cultivating awareness of the Middle Pillar of the Tree of Life in his book by that name (see figure 14). I present Regardie's exercise here in slightly modified form to accommodate our energy studies.

In this exercise, you will vibrate some divine Hebrew names as you draw energy down. These are not "mantras," but words of power. Regardie insisted that these words were "vibratory formulas" that can put your mind on the proper "frequency" for magick. While this makes it easy to avoid any kind of religious implications, I also think it is important to remember that these words are, after all, names of God—not necessarily in a theological sense, but as a concept of the highest and most sublime energy in the universe.

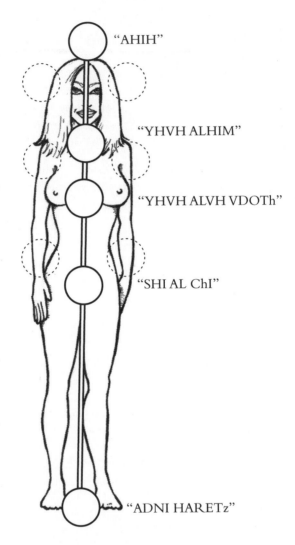

Figure 14. The Middle Pillar

Mastering the Middle Pillar

1. Sit in a comfortable position, lie down flat, or stand.
2. Enter a magick trance.
3. Imagine that your breath is coming into and out of your crown chakra. This may seem tenuous at first, but don't worry. The impression will soon strengthen.

4. Continue to breathe into your crown chakra. Visualize a sphere or star of bright white shining just above your head, about the size of a grapefruit, in the region of your breathing. Imagine light pouring out of it as if it were a small Sun.

5. Inhale, concentrating intently on the breath filling up the star above your head. As you exhale, vibrate the word "AHIH" (eh-hay-ee-ay). Watch and feel the star growing in brilliance. Feel this energy as mild or even extreme sexual ecstasy, just as when you were drawing it up through your sex organs. Repeat this process five times.

6. Relax for a few moments and feel the energy pulsing above your head.

7. Exhale, and imagine that you are pushing a shaft of white light down through your head from the star above you, to your throat. Begin breathing energy down the shaft into your throat, always beginning at the star above your head. Continue to feel this as a sensual pleasure.

8. Visualize a second sphere or star in the center of your throat. Inhale, concentrating intently on the energy descending into your throat. As you exhale, vibrate the words "IHVH ALHIM" (yay-ho-vaoh ay-lo-heem). Watch and feel the star brighten. Repeat this process five times.

9. Relax and feel the energy pulsing through your head and throat.

10. Exhale, and push the shaft of white light from the star in your throat down to the area around your heart and solar plexus. Breathe energy down the shaft into your throat and down to your chest, always beginning at the star above your head.

11. Visualize a third sphere or star in the center of your chest. Inhale, concentrating intently on the energy descending into your chest. As you exhale, vibrate the words "IHVH ALVH VDOTh" (yay-ho-vaoh ay-lo-ah vay-dah-awth). The star should become more brilliant as you do this. Repeat this process five times.

12. Relax and observe your body, noticing any changes, and feel the pulsation of the energy.

13. Exhale, and push the shaft of white light through your chest from the star above you, down to your pelvic area. Breathe energy down the shaft into your throat, down to your chest, and all the way down to your pelvis, always beginning at the star above your head.

14. Visualize a fourth sphere or star around your genitals. Inhale, concentrating intently on the energy descending into your genitals. As you exhale, vibrate the words "SDI AL ChI" (shaw-die el ch-eye). Feel the star growing in brilliance as you do this. Repeat this process five times.

15. Relax and feel this powerful flow of energy.

16. Exhale, and push the shaft of white light down through your genitals from the star above you, to your feet. Breathe energy down the shaft into your throat to your chest, through your genitals, and down to your feet, always beginning at the star above your head.

17. Visualize a fifth sphere or star around your feet. Inhale, concentrating intently on the energy descending into your feet. As you exhale, vibrate the words "ADNI HARTz" (ad-on-eye ha-ar-ets). Feel the star growing in brilliance as you do this. Repeat this process five times.

18. Relax and observe your body once again, noticing whatever is happening there, and feel the radiating energy.

19. Maintaining the downward flow as much as possible, focus your attention back on the star above your head. Exhale, and push a ball of light and energy out of the star above your head and down the left side of your body to the star beneath your feet. Inhale and bring it back up your right side to the star above your head, forming a circle of light around you. Repeat this five times, or until it seems solid.

20. Exhale, and bring a ball of light down the front of your body to the star beneath your feet. Inhale and bring it back up the rear of your body to the star above your head, forming another circle of light. Repeat this process five times.

21. Relax for a few moments and feel all of these pathways of energy as well as you can.

22. Focus your attention on the star beneath your feet. Inhale and bring a spiraling shaft of light swirling up around your body to the star above your head. While exhaling, visualize a fireworks-like explosion of light that rains gently down upon you and is collected into the star beneath your feet. Repeat this process five times.

23. Enjoy this energy for as long as you wish.

24. Record your experience in your journal.

Image, Energy, and Inspiration

The three essential keys for success in any magick are image, energy, and inspiration. Other authors have made similar observations, calling them imagination, will, and gnosis.[42] You must formulate a clear idea or image of what you want, attach great energy to it, and seek higher consciousness in an altered state to bring about the result.

This is the essence of all successful practical magick, whatever form these components eventually take. A brief analysis of any magical operation shows that these concepts are universal. Sex magick contains so much power because you automatically create huge amounts of energy and inspiration just by engaging in the loving connection of the sex act. All you need to do is add the image of what you want to conjure up an absolutely perfect act of magick.

Your thoughts during sex are truly powerful, because they are images of that toward which you are directing magical forces, whether you are aware of what you are doing or not. In truly passionate sex, this happens automatically, without you even being aware of it. That is why so many great contributors to culture—artists, scientists, or politicians—are also passionate lovers. The power of sexual energy charged with the purpose of accomplishing great things in life is nearly unstoppable. Many people also unconsciously use this power to control their partners, by directing their sexual force to dominate and captivate them. This is, of course, not a healthy use of this energy, as it drags the practitioner into unhealthy places.

In some Gnostic ideas about sex, the Holy Spirit is a combination of the male and the female—a metaphysical ecstasy of sexual union in which God is made manifest. This is the great fountain of inspiration necessary for all magick. This inspiration is inherent in the love felt between the two coupled in the sex act, whether the coupling is hetero- or homosexual.

What you think about during sex—combined with sexual passion and your ecstatic, divine connection with your partner—creates a magical child. At orgasm, you impress your will upon the universe. It is an extremely powerful creative moment. Your dreams and desires are imprinted on consciousness at a very deep level in orgasm, rivaling any other peak experience in life. As all your senses lapse into ecstasy, you open a gateway of manifestation. And that toward which you direct this power will come to fruition, as the energy form created by the sex act seeks a method of grounding itself in actualization.

The female operant is as capable of formulating, creating, and guiding the career of this magical energy form as the male. It is really only in the writings of Crowley and his heirs that we find statements about women being incapable of accomplishing this work on their own. Crowley's stance was really due to the inherent sexism of the Victorian age, however, and a lack of understanding that the real biological basis of life is an equal exchange of genetic and spiritual material from both mother and father into the life of the child.

Crowley says that the role of woman is "...to arrange and to adjust all Things that exist in their proper Sphere, but not to create or transcend." He seems to feel that women are practically unable to accomplish the heroic path of the Great Work on their own, or to conduct sexual magick effectively. But consider that water is the force that created the Grand Canyon. Water is one of the most powerful substances and forces known. It is a nearly universal solvent; almost everything dissolves in water. In hurricanes and tidal waves, it destroys wantonly. In rains, it nourishes the world. If woman's archetype is water, I hardly think this is something to scoff at. By contrast, fire, usually considered "man's formula," is pure destruction when undirected, yet carefully wielded fire has created civilization. The same can easily be said of water. No matter how you look at it, women are as powerful as men metaphysically, and, even if their methods are somewhat different, their power should never be questioned.

There is a Gnostic myth in which the goddess Sophia hides her power within humanity to prevent the demiurge Ialdabaoth (perhaps equivalent to Jehovah) from accessing it. This power is the force of the true highest God, the Monad. Kundalini Shakti is essentially the same concept in Indian Tantric philosophy. This power is the source of all creativity, all human thought, all life. Through it, we create our perceptions of the world. Through it, we become sexual sorcerers.

As you engage in ecstatic sexual activities, you stir up all of the subtle energies that course through your body, most particularly the divine power at your core. This Sophia, or Shakti, is in your sexual fluids, in your blood, your breath—you are that power. Once you have released the blocks that stop the flow of this energy, it imbues your sexual activities with the force of the divine seed within you. But you can only unlock this power fully when you have freed yourself from energy blockages.

DNA, Procreation, and Magick

As we all know, from the vantage point of modern medical science, pregnancy results from a sperm cell reaching an egg that is ripe for fertilization. Thanks to research by Watson and Frick into the structure of DNA, we also know that this process of fertilization entails a precise 50/50 exchange of DNA from the mother and the father. In the late 1800s, however, it was still possible to fantasize that it was the man who gave life to the fetus with his activating sperm, while the female egg remained relatively inert in the process. While it was understood that the female somehow contributed some of her biological essence to the operation, so that the child might in some way resemble her, most believed it was the man who really "gave life" to the child. It was under this illusion that most sex-magical literature was constructed. In Crowley's tarot image The Devil, for instance, a pair of testicles containing human forms appears at the bottom of the card, implying that these little people will just pop out inside the woman and grow into babies.

The facts of reproduction as we know them today are quite different. In the testicles and the ovaries, the process of myosis creates a collection of partial human cells that contain only half of the chromosomes necessary for the creation of a fetus. When a sperm cell reaches an egg cell, it releases its DNA into the nucleus of the egg, where it pairs with the DNA of the egg. Physiologically, the male sperm is inert without the DNA of the female egg. Likewise, the egg is inert without the sperm. It is only in their connection and mingling of genetic material that new life emerges—new life that contains equal parts of both parents.

The same is energetically true in sex magick. It is the mingling energies of both parties that create the "magical child." There is no reason to suppose that the female is any less significant in the operation than the male. Nor is there any reason to assume that two same-sex partners of either gender should be excluded from creating "magical children." Of course, these may differ slightly from those of their heterosexual counterparts, but that is more a subject for experimentation than speculation.

There are autoerotic magical practices that do not require a physical partner of any kind. In these operations there is always a partner of a spiritual nature, however—a god form, an archetype of some sort, an elemental being, or an astral form vivified by passion into a real and powerful sexual energy form of its own. We will explore a number of these cases in the coming chapters. For now, experiment with building up your own sexual energy to a peak of magical power.

Magical Chastity—First Type

For the next week or so, observe chastity in its most usual sense. Make every effort to avoid sexuality in deed and even thought. Should any sexual thoughts come into your mind—for instance, if by chance you see an attractive person walking by—immediately redirect this passion to further understanding your True Will and gaining the Knowledge and Conversation of the Holy Guardian Angel. Keep a record of your successes in your journal. Take special care to observe your state throughout the week and keep notes about how this kind of chastity makes you feel.

CHAPTER 4

Building Sex Power and Orgasmic Energy

I am the secret Serpent coiled about to spring: in my coiling there is joy. If I lift up my head, I and my Nuit are one. If I droop down mine head, and shoot forth venom, then is rapture of the earth, and I and the earth are one.

—*Liber AL vel Legis, II, 26*

Now we approach the heart of the matter. There are three essential sexual skills you must cultivate to become a sexual sorcerer:

- The ability to awaken and direct your body's ecstatic sexual energies at will
- The ability to have an orgasm when you want one
- The ability not to have an orgasm when you don't want one

To begin actively directing your sexual energy toward magical purposes, you must explore your own sexual energy system so you can begin to understand it intimately and consciously.

Most of us have at least some blocks and fears related to our sexuality. These limit the full power of our inherent sex force. You cannot fully acquire the three essential skills of the sexual sorcerer until at least some of these blocks have been removed. Ideally, you should eradicate all of these fears and blocks to become truly free to experience real sexual bliss. This bliss is your true power; in it, you are really connected to your divine inner nature.

Our culture sends extremely mixed messages about sex to children early in their development. On the one hand, we are tantalized with ubiquitous sexualized images—particularly of women—in all forms of media. On the other hand, we are subconsciously instructed that our own sexuality and sexual feelings are somehow inappropriate. Sex is not discussed at most dinner tables and, if it comes up at all, it is usually accompanied by blushing, giggling, and discomfort, even in relatively mature adults. Parents are uneasy in varying degrees when they discuss sex with their children. When children become sexually active, their parents either discourage them, or tease or embarrass them about their sexual feelings. With so little guidance, our early sexual experiences are almost always tinged with a sense of doubt or shame. This is particularly true of women. I have talked to countless women who spent their teenage years feeling thoroughly horrified by their body, and by sexuality in general.

Men, on the other hand, are often filled with doubts about their ability to perform and please women. They doubt the size, shape, and staying power of their penises, although they usually love them despite these doubts. In fact, I think that all men secretly bestow upon their penises the same sort of love and worship that most bestow upon their god. They seek to enlarge it in the minds of others and wish ardently that it was more universally adored. Some women may view their vaginas in the same way, but I have known several who seem to dislike their sex organs, fearing odor and monthly blood. Men often contribute to these fears, wrinkling their noses or outright cringing at the thought of menstruation and making insensitive comments. A woman's sex organs deserve adoration. They are a center of the holiest delights, and the gateway through which we all enter life.

In our culture, we hardly ever discuss the real development of either emotional or physical sexual functionality, even in sex-education classes. Sexual dysfunction of one sort or another plagues many of both sexes. I myself used to have a problem with premature ejaculation when I was younger. Luckily, the techniques given in this chapter enabled me to become a powerful sexual sorcerer. Many people, however, do not fully enjoy sex and don't experience powerful and transformative orgasmic ecstasies even if their sex organs function properly. Even those who escape the most obvious sexual traumas carry around some sexual and emotional wounds that scar their intimate relationships and create challenges in connecting with lovers on an interpersonal level. And this certainly affects their ability to direct their sex forces magically.

Sexual dysfunction is rampant in our culture in both men and women. Many women, young and old, lose their sexual interest and sex drive completely. While this is nothing new, it is just beginning to receive cultural attention. Wilhelm Reich, who was aware of this problem eighty years ago, called it "the Emotional Plague." Reich felt that men and women both suffered from this affliction. Premature ejaculation, erectile problems, lack of sensation, too much sensation, lack of self-lubrication, inability to achieve orgasm—all are huge problems in our culture that affect the quality of sex for both genders. Pharmaceutical companies and medical professionals make a killing selling cure-all pills to those who experience them.

Reich, Character Armor, and Orgone

Wilhelm Reich began his career working in a free clinic in Vienna. As a student of Sigmund Freud, he was naturally interested in the libido and the connection of sexual feelings to neuroses. When Reich discovered that the vast majority of his patients were suffering directly from some sort of sexual dysfunction, he began to formulate a theory about the psychological importance of fully functional orgasmic release.

In Reich's theory of orgasm, release involves not only achieving orgasm. It requires the complete release of the tension created by the desire. He describes this in somewhat mystical terms as a sort of massive pleasure that obliterates any sense of self. "The mystical ideas of innumerable religions, the belief in the beyond, the doctrine of the transmigration of the soul, etc., derive, without exception, from cosmic longing; and functionally, the cosmic yearning is anchored in the expressive movements of the orgasm reflex."[43] Reich felt that orgasm should be a complete temporary loss of ego boundaries—a flowing of your consciousness into your partner's and the universal energy flow.

Reich soon began to move beyond Freud's theories, developing his own concepts of "character armor" and the universal life energy. He called this life energy *orgone* to clearly illustrate its relationship to orgasm. Reich's orgone is similar to prana or chi, though he showed little knowledge of these concepts in his own writings. He came upon his idea of orgone through a series of laboratory experiments in which he believed himself to have discovered *bions*, the individual units of life force. Unfortunately, Reich ran afoul of the A.M.A. and the pharmaceutical companies in the '50s, and much of his very interesting work has been hidden from the public eye.

Reich felt that orgone energy should flow freely through the body, enlivening cells, supplying energy and inspiration, and flowing between sexual partners in ecstatic orgasmic release. He felt, however, that the vast majority of humans were incapable of such release. Reich found a characteristic muscular tension in his orgasmically dysfunctional patients—their character armor or emotional rigidity—that followed certain definite patterns with a segmental arrangement. He noted that this seven-part segmental arrangement of tension resembled the structure and function of ringed worms or other lower forms of life, indicating that it reflected something primal within the body. These seven character-armor segments are not, however, related to the skeletal system, although they may mirror the spinal cord, which is segmented, and the nerve plexuses attached to it. Modern yogis have compared the chakras to the nerve plexuses in a similar way. In fact, the seven chakras and Reich's seven character-armor rings seem to correspond well with each other and the major nerve plexuses.

These segments are like rings of tension that squeeze around the body, preventing the orgone, or life energy, from moving freely. The natural flow of energy is vertical, from feet to head, but Reich's character-armor rings encircle the body horizontally, blocking the natural flow of energy and inhibiting the natural functioning of our basic sexual energy. Figure 15 portrays this in some detail.

It is interesting to compare these character-armor rings with the chakras of the Indian yogis. Although there are a few differences, the similarities are very remarkable, considering that Reich worked from observation rather than trying to create something that corresponded to Eastern metaphysics. In fact, Reich's energy flow closely mirrors the flow of kundalini—the magical sex force essential to sexual metaphysics. His analysis of these blockages, which are essentially identical to the closed chakras awakened in yogic practices, can help you understand the blockages that limit your own sex-magical force. According to Reich, your characteristic tensions, doubts, fears, and neurotic habit-patterns inhibit the natural flow of your vitality and power, keeping your chakras closed and your essence concealed.

Every neurotic tendency that you have, whether sexual or not, derives from this emotional armor. Everything that makes you feel uncomfortable, pushes your boundaries, or otherwise makes you tense is armoring that keeps you from experiencing the free flow of bliss, impairs your sexuality, and impacts your enjoyment of life in general. Because we have all suffered some damage relating to sex in our lives, these blockages become particularly evident in the sexual arena.

Reich created a number of techniques for releasing these tensions—from talk therapy, to massage-like treatments, to movement therapy. He even developed orgone accumulator machines that got him into a lot

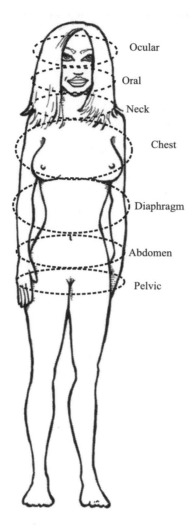

Figure 15. Reich's character armor

of trouble. There are quite a few Reichian therapists still practicing today, however, as well as modern developments like "bioenergetics" that are based on his ideas. Here, we will look at a number of ways in which you can familiarize yourself with your own blockages, and begin to release some, perhaps all, of your armoring. The key to this process is really a desire to be free, a desire to feel true ecstasy, and the commitment to look fearlessly at the truth of your present condition. It is easy to pretend that you are perfectly fine, that there is nothing wrong. But the true sexual sorcerer is never satisfied with self-perpetuated illusions.

Learn to treat your sexual energy like a power line. To increase the amplitude and frequency of the energy coursing through you, try putting as much energy through your system as possible. At times, this may be painful—when love is lost or you are somehow insulted—but if you moderate that pain, you also moderate your joy. We all armor ourselves, at least a little, to protect ourselves from potential pain. You must remove this armor to experience real pleasure.

Try to remove all barriers; allow yourself to be harmed and to feel true ecstasy. Remember, only your false self is at risk. Your true self can never be harmed, and is always in ecstasy. When you let yourself truly experience everything, the false becomes more apparent, and you get closer to your Holy Guardian Angel and your self. This is the key concept of Eastern Tantra. By opening up to experience and removing your inhibitions and fears, you begin to comprehend the totality. You slip between the elements of experience into the transcendent.

You begin this process by approaching your blockages directly. One of the most productive ways to begin to work through your energy blockages and get energy flowing through you on a higher level is to take up a regular practice of yoga or the martial arts. These practices will clear and exhilarate you, and get you into shape at the same time. Being in excellent physical condition will help you sexually. Good conditioning can extend your sexual experiences passionately, and make you a more attractive and magnetic mate. Find a class immediately, and go two to five times a week.

Your Character Armor

Remember all those questions you asked yourself in our earlier exercises? Well now you can apply that work to an understanding of some of your own emotional armoring. You may even wish to repeat the exercise, this time paying particular attention to where in your body you feel different emotions at different times, and how these emotions affect your well-being.

For instance, notice where in your body you characteristically hold tension, and where you hold tension when facing different sorts of challenges in life. Do these tensions correspond to Reichian character armor and the Hindu chakras? Observe these blockages throughout the day for several days, and record your observations in your journal.

Once you have identified a few places where you are characteristically holding onto tension, you can begin to explore the fears and old pains that may be lodged in these areas, either in a magick trance or just casually. Once you have located these tensions, begin to release them with the next six exercises.

These exercises may be traumatic if you have severe armoring, neuroses, and blockages. It may be wise to consult a psychological professional before doing these exercises. If you know that you have a history of serious psychological problems, please seek out a therapist.

Most of us are at least mildly armored in all places, so try to explore all of the releasing techniques. Remember, if there is an area you want to avoid, it probably means this area is blocked, and you may feel uncomfortable releasing this block. Achieving release is a challenging project that requires a significant amount of personal courage. But sexual sorcerers know that courage is essential to success in any endeavor.

The first exercise gives you simple little movements that can help you clear away some of your habitual body armor and discover those areas in which you are blocked. If you find any of these exercises either too trivial or too difficult for you to conduct, you can rest assured that you are dealing with an area in which you are armored.

Releasing Body Tension

1. Stand with your feet at shoulder-width apart, your head erect, and your arms at your sides. Bend your knees slightly, so that they are not locked. Imagine that a string attached to the top of your head is pulling your whole body upward, so that your back is straight and erect. Tuck your pelvis forward to support your back.
2. Release your eyes and face: Scrunch your whole face in like a raisin and then open your whole face wide, opening your eyes and leaving your mouth agape. Repeat this several times.
3. Release your mouth and jaw: Smile widely, then frown. Repeat several times. Roll your jaw around several times, then repeat the whole process.
4. Release your neck: Turn your head from side to side. Drop your head to your chest and roll it halfway around on each side so that your chin moves to each shoulder. Tilt your head forward and back. Repeat several times.

5. Release your chest: Clasp your hands behind your back and raise
   them up straight behind you, spreading your shoulders back.
   Lean your whole body forward and back a few times.
6. Release your diaphragm and abdomen: Spread your arms to the
   side, raising them to shoulder height. Pivot from side to side,
   swinging your arms in wide arcs.
7. Release your pelvis: Roll your pelvis in a figure-eight pattern,
   first to one side and then the other.
8. Record your experiences in your journal.

The next exercise approaches this tension release from a slightly more
metaphysical perspective. You can use it to pull energy through your
chakras. This will start the process of clearing and engaging them more
fully.

Breathing through Your Chakras

1. Sit or lie down in a comfortable place.
2. Enter a magick trance.
3. Breathe in slowly, drawing in energy using your perineum. As
   you inhale, move this vibration of energy from you perineum up
   into your sex organs, your Svadisthana chakra.
4. On the same inhalation, continue to breathe in and draw your
   energy up through each of your chakras: the Manipura chakra
   located at your belly, then the Anahata at the center of your
   chest, then the Vishuddha at your throat, the Ajna between your
   eyes, and the Sahasrara at the crown of your head. Make sure that
   you really feel energy flowing up through each of these chakras.
   Feel this energy through the whole circuit of your body, from
   your front all the way back to your spine. If you are unsure about
   any of them, go back to the descriptions on page 93 and locate
   them clearly. It may take a few tries before you can make it
   through all the chakras in a single breath. Just keep trying until
   you get the timing and sensations down.
5. Each chakra may present you with a different feeling. Observe
   these, but don't be concerned if you notice blocks or strange
   feelings. You may not feel anything in certain chakras, or you may
   have many blockages in you, or you may find it difficult to pass
   the energy through certain chakras. Be patient. This exercise and
   the next will help to open you up.

6. When you reach the crown of your head, or run out of breath, reverse the process, sending the energy down through each chakra, and finally out through your perineum at the base of your spine.

7. When you become proficient at this, you will be able to send this energy through each of your chakras easily. You should feel a profound sense of pleasure doing this exercise, once you get it. As the energy reaches your crown, or Sahasrara chakra, you may begin to feel as if your body disappears, or as if a small explosion takes place inside you. This is good; but remember to send the energy back downward. Continue this pattern for several breaths.

8. Record your experiences in your journal.

The next exercise helps you open up, explore, and clear away some of the blocks in your chakras. If you experience any significant emotional strain or lack of feeling in any of these chakras as you perform this exercise, stand up and move around, twisting and bending your body as described above to release blockages. Try to move and open the particular area of your body that feels blocked.

It may help you to focus on a color for each chakra while doing this, imagining each chakra as a small sphere of the appropriate color. The popular New Age colors for the chakras will work just fine. They are as follows:

Red	Muladhara (chakra)
Orange	Svadhisthana (chakra)
Yellow	Manipura(chakra)
Green	Anahata (chakra)
Blue	Vishudda (chakra)
Indigo	Ajna (chakra)
Violet or white	Sahasrara (chakra)

Don't feel confined to these colors. If some other color, shape, or feeling seems more appropriate to you, explore it.

Breathing in Chakra Energy

1. Sit or lie down in a comfortable place.
2. Enter a magick trance.
3. Begin your sexual-energy breathing. Breathe in and out through your Muladhara chakra, but this time, attempt to contain the

energy within the area around your perineum. Focus exclusively on the Muladhara region. Create in your mind a set of imaginary hands that reach inside you and pull open this area. Feel a sensation as if you were opening an orifice. Breathe all the way into yourself, feeling the energy from your perineum to the base of your spine. Feel any emotions that seem to come up in this area; be with them non-judgmentally and let them flow.

4. Shift your awareness to your Svadhisthana chakra at the base of your genitals. Begin to breathe in and out through your Svadhisthana region. You may gently contract this area if it helps you to focus as you breathe in. This may take a few moments to master, but should not be too difficult. If energy seems to be flowing down to your Muladhara, or up into your belly, gently coax it to stay in the Svadhisthana region. Breathe in and out through your Svadhisthana for several minutes, observing the character of the sensation. Each chakra has its own distinct feeling. Create in your mind a set of imaginary hands that reach inside you and pull open this area. Feel a sensation as if you were opening an orifice. Breathe all the way into yourself, feeling the energy moving into you from the base of your sex organs and flowing back to your spine, sending sensation through you. Feel any emotions that seem to come up in this area; be with them non-judgmentally and let them flow. If thoughts, emotions, or images arise, let them happen, and let them go.

5. Breathe through each of your chakras in the same manner, until you have become familiar with and opened all seven. Be sure to allow the sensation of each chakra to fill the whole region, from the front of your body to your spine.

6. Record your experiences in your journal.

You can also balance and clear yourself through the two hemispheres of your body, right and left. Alternate-nostril breathing offers a simple and excellent way to balance out these two hemispheres. You may need to blow your nose before you perform this exercise. Remember to use long, slow, complete breaths.

Alternate-Nostril Breathing

1. Close your right nostril with your thumb, and exhale completely through your left nostril. Then inhale through your left nostril.

2. Seal your left nostril with your middle finger, and exhale through your right nostril.
3. Keeping your left nostril sealed, inhale through your right nostril.
4. Seal your right nostril, and exhale your breath completely through your left nostril once again. This is one cycle; it can be repeated for as long as you like.
5. Record your experiences in your journal.

Ten minutes of regular alternate-nostril breathing should balance you very well. You can also combine this with breath-retention techniques to enhance the energetic clearing. You can use the four-fold breath: Breathe in for a count of four, hold your breath in for a count of four, let it out for a count of four, and hold it out for a count of four. You can also use the traditional yogic technique: breathe in for four counts, hold for sixteen counts, and release for eight counts. This can also be expanded to 6:24:12, 8:32:16, and so on.

The next two exercises are designed to help you bring a powerful charge of kundalini energy into your body. Once you have cleared some of your inner blockages, try to increase the power of the energy flowing into you by using one or both of them. You may immediately feel the flow of kundalini, or it may take several sessions. In either case, once you start doing these exercises, you may notice a number of strange energy surges in your body, even when you are not using the techniques. You may also have troubling experiences if you use this technique before you are ready.

Arousing Kundalini

1. Sit or lie down in a comfortable place.
2. Breathe in and out a few times to relax, and enter a magick trance.
3. Spend a few minutes doing alternate-nostril breathing as described above.
4. Begin with a few minutes of breathing energy up through all of your chakras. Really feel the energy move in and out.
5. After a few minutes, inhale deeply, contracting your perineum and drawing the energy up through your chakras. Hold your breath for as long as you comfortably can, continuing to draw energy up through your whole energy body.

6. As you exhale completely, hold your perineum contracted, keeping the energy inside. You may feel it sinking, but don't let it out.

7. When you have exhaled completely, hold your breath out, keeping your perineum contracted as before. And as you are holding your breath out, draw in your abdomen, as if you were trying to get your navel to touch your spine. You will feel an inner sucking sensation. As you do this, suck energy up into your spine as if it were a straw.

8. This may make you shake after a few seconds. Keep this sucking sensation going as you contract your perineum and abdomen. You will know that it is working when a tingle of energy begins to move up your spine. If it starts to make your eyes tense or burn, tuck your chin to your chest. Hold for as long as possible, then inhale, raise your head, and continue to draw energy up your spine.

9. Breathe in again, drawing more energy up into your chakras through your contracted perineum. Return to step 4 above and repeat the process, until your whole body is literally swimming with energy. Try beginning with five breaths, then expand to more when you are comfortable.

10. Record your experiences in your journal.

The following is an even simpler technique that you may find equally effective.

Arousing Kundalini in Your Belly Cauldron

1. Sit or lie down in a comfortable place.
2. Breathe in and out a few times to relax, and enter a magick trance.
3. Spend a few minutes doing alternate-nostril breathing, as described above.
4. Continue with a few minutes of breathing energy up through all of your chakras. Really feel the energy move in and out.
5. On an inhalation, draw up some energy from your root into your belly, while imagining that the breath energy you are drawing in from above is also going down into your belly.
6. Hold your breath, imagining that these two energies combine in your belly cauldron and heat up, then push them down into your

Muladhara, or base, chakra, to awaken the kundalini. Allow the energy to rush back up your spine if it will. Repeat as many times as you feel comfortable.

7. Record your experiences in your journal.

Energized Ritual

The same ecstatic energy that we have been exploring can turn even the simplest ritual into a divine union of amazing proportions. The following are some simple instructions for directing this energy in the Lesser Ritual of the Pentagram that we explored earlier in chapter 4. There are many variations on this and other rituals in the literature. This same idea can also be applied in the Thelemic Star Ruby ritual and other rituals.[44]

Energetic Lesser Ritual of the Pentagram

1. Enter a magick trance.
2. You may start by breathing through your chakras, and/or arousing kundalini through one of the above techniques in order to get the flow of energy moving through your body. Focus on moving a charge of ecstatic energy to your crown chakra, your personal Qabalistic Kether.
3. Stand facing east.
4. Begin breathing into your crown chakra, visualizing a globe of white light burning like a star directly above your head. Feel the ecstasy of this as palpably as possible. Raise your right hand above your head, and draw a shaft of light down into your head from the star. Visualize a shaft of white light rising vertically from the globe above your head to infinity. Touch your forehead, vibrating the word "AThH" (aw-tay).
5. Inhale deeply and feel the globe above your head burning with intensity as it sends light down into your head. Exhale slowly, and continue to draw the shaft of light down with your hand to your groin area, vibrating the word "MLKVTh" (mall-kooth). Visualize the vertical shaft of white light descending all the way to another globe beneath your feet, and onward, through the center of the Earth, to infinity. Feel this as a descent of bliss into your body.

6. Touch your right shoulder, vibrating "VGBVRH" (vay-geh-boo-rah). Breathe into your shoulder, visualizing another globe shining where you are touching your shoulder, and a shaft of white light extending horizontally to your right, and on to infinity.

7. Touch your left shoulder, vibrating "VGDVLH" (vay-ged-joo-lah). Breathe into your shoulder, visualizing another globe shining where you are touching your shoulder, and a shaft of white light extending horizontally to your left, and on to infinity.

8. Bring both your hands to your heart. Begin breathing energy from all four points (above your head, beneath your feet, and at your left and right shoulders) into your heart, forming a sphere of brilliant light and energy. This should feel quite ecstatic. When it becomes almost unbearable, vibrate "LOVLM" (lay-oh-law-um), causing the ecstasy to double or triple until you are nearly destroyed with joy.

9. Interlace your fingers. Stand at the center of the blazing cross of white light that extends to the ends of the universe and vibrate "AMN" (Amen). As you say this, see and feel the globe of light at your heart growing to fill the whole magical circle, so that you are in a sphere of divine energy.

10. Go to the east. Send energy from your heart up through your arm as you exhale, tracing a banishing Earth pentagram. As you trace, visualize a blue flame forming the pentagram in the air before you. Be aware that you are setting in motion forces that will keep all hostile influences from your circle. Inhale deeply, drawing energy down from the globe above your head. Visualize the letters "YHVH" coming down into your body with the energy. Send the energy and the letters all the way down to the globe beneath your feet. As you exhale, send the energy up and outward as you vibrate "YHVH" (yay-ho-vaoh) using the Sign of the Enterer (see figure 16, page 121). Visualize the energy bursting through and past the pentagram, blasting away all negative energy as it fills a quarter of the entire universe. Give the Sign of Silence as you inhale and withdraw the extended energy. Behind the pentagram, an amorphous shape of energy should remain. This will become the archangel at the appropriate time.

11. Pierce the center of the pentagram. Send some of your energy out of your body as you exhale, tracing a line of white light

around your circle as you move to the south (to the point that will become the center of the next pentagram).

12. Inhale deeply, drawing energy from the globe above your head into your heart. Send energy from your heart up through your arm as you exhale, tracing a banishing Earth pentagram. As you trace, visualize a blue flame forming the pentagram in the air before you. Be aware that you are setting in motion forces that will keep all hostile influences from your circle. Inhale deeply, drawing energy down from the globe above your head. Visualize the letters "ADNI" coming down into your body with the energy. Send the energy and the letters all the way down to the globe beneath your feet. As you exhale, send the energy up and outward as you vibrate "ADNI" (ad-on-eye) using the Sign of the Enterer. Visualize the energy bursting through and past the pentagram, blasting away all negative energy as it fills a quarter of the entire universe. Give the Sign of Silence as you inhale and withdraw the extended energy. Behind the pentagram, an amorphous shape of energy should remain. This will become the archangel at the appropriate time

13. Pierce the center of the pentagram. Send some of your energy out of your body as you exhale, tracing a line of white light as you move to the west (to the point that will become the center of the next pentagram).

14. Inhale deeply, drawing energy from the globe above your head into your heart. Send energy from your heart up through your arm as you exhale, tracing a banishing Earth pentagram. As you trace, visualize a blue flame forming the pentagram in the air before you. Be aware that you are setting in motion forces that will keep all hostile influences from your circle. Inhale deeply, drawing energy down from the globe above your head. Visualize the letters "AHIH" coming down into your body with the energy. Send the energy and the letters all the way down to the globe beneath your feet. As you exhale, send the energy up and outward as you vibrate "AHIH" (eh-hay-ee-ay) using the Sign of the Enterer. Visualize the energy bursting through and past the pentagram, blasting away all negative energy as it fills a quarter of the entire universe. Give the Sign of Silence as you inhale and withdraw the extended energy. Behind the pentagram, an amorphous shape of energy should remain. This will become the archangel at the appropriate time.

15. Pierce the center of the pentagram. Send some of your energy out of your body as you exhale, tracing a line of white light as you move to the north (to the point that will become the center of the next pentagram).

16. Inhale deeply, drawing energy from the globe above your head into your heart. Send energy from your heart up through your arm as you exhale, tracing a banishing Earth pentagram. As you trace, visualize a blue flame forming the pentagram in the air before you. Be aware that you are setting in motion forces that will keep all hostile influences from your circle. Inhale deeply, drawing energy down from the globe above your head. Visualize the letters "AGLA" coming down into your body with the energy. Send the energy and the letters all the way down to the globe beneath your feet. As you exhale, send the energy up and outward as you vibrate "AGLA" (ah-geh-lah) using the Sign of the Enterer. Visualize the energy bursting through and past the pentagram, blasting away all negative energy as it fills a quarter of the entire universe. Give the Sign of Silence as you inhale and withdraw the extended energy. Behind the pentagram, an amorphous shape of energy should remain. This will become the archangel at the appropriate time.

17. Pierce the center of the pentagram. Send some of your energy out of your body as you exhale, tracing a line of white light as you move to the east. Complete the circle by finishing the line in the center of the first pentagram (where you began).

18. Stand facing east, with your arms outstretched in a cross at shoulder level. Inhale deeply, drawing down energy from the globe above into your heart. Say "Before me 'RPAL' (ra-phay-al)." As you intone the name of the archangel, visualize him materializing behind your pentagram. With each syllable, his shape should become more manifest. Repeat with the other archangels, saying, "behind me 'GBRIAL' (gah-bree-al), on my right hand 'MIKAL' (mee-kah-al), on my left hand 'AURIAL' (or-ee-al)." Observe the energy in and about you, saying, "About me flame the pentagrams, and in the column shines the six-rayed star."

19. Repeat steps four through nine.

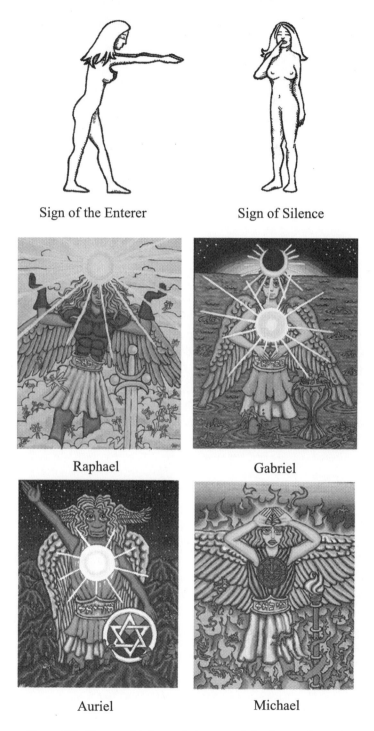

Sign of the Enterer   Sign of Silence

Raphael   Gabriel

Auriel   Michael

Figure 16. Signs and telesmatic images of the four archangels

Magical Chastity—Second Type

As you become more proficient with your sexual energy, try observing magical chasitity in its second sense for a week or so. That is to say, you can explore sexuality either through energetic work, masturbation, or sex with a partner, but make every effort to avoid genital orgasm. Explore and move your sexual energy throughout your body, but do not allow yourself to have a genital orgasm for at least a week. The more often you excite yourself sexually, the more powerful this experience will be. There are many potential benefits to this practice, as you will see.

It is very easy to succumb to orgasm when in the embrace of your lover. You may require a lot of practice to really control the orgasm reflex if you are a man or a particularly orgasmic woman. It may be best simply to abstain from sexual relations with your partner for this week. Some partners may be disappointed or even insulted if you don't achieve orgasm. They may feel that you are not really interested in them. If this occurs, just communicate exactly what you are doing, and explain that it is part of an attempt to understand and explore your sexual energy.

As you practice this second type of magical chastity, continue to direct all of your sexual energy toward further understanding your True Will and gaining the Knowledge and Conversation of the Holy Guardian Angel. Keep a record of your success in your journal, observing your state throughout the week. Keep notes about how this kind of chastity makes you feel, both physically and emotionally.

The following exercise is key to establishing control over your orgasmic reflex. While this practice is very simple, its ramifications are profound. If you are a man, you will be able resist ejaculation for as long as you want and to experience repeated orgasmic delight within a single sex act by pulling back at the very last moment before ejaculation. You will also be able to extend the feelings of orgasm over a much longer period of time whether you are a man or a woman. Once you have mastered this incredibly powerful technique, you may find regular genital orgasm less enticing than these inner whole-body orgasmic experiences.

Autoerotic Energetic Practice

1. To begin, simply start masturbating. You may wish to somehow separate this masturbation into a magical context through preliminary ritual or meditation, but this is not really necessary.

2. Masturbate until you are just about to have an orgasm, until you are just at the "point of no return," say 90–95 percent of the way there. But do not yield to orgasm. Instead, contract your perineum as in the previous exercises, and draw that highly charged sexual energy up into your body. You can draw it up through all of your chakras, or you can draw it up into a particular chakra, perhaps one that you feel is slightly blocked. You can circulate the energy in your body as in the Lesser Heavenly Circle exercise (see page 96), or you can use one of the kundalini-arousing breathing techniques (see pages 98–100).
3. Once you are calmed and the energy has been usefully directed, you may resume masturbation.
4. Repeat this process several times, avoiding orgasm, of course, if you are practicing the second form of magical chastity.
5. Record your experiences in your journal.

Once you have become somewhat adept at this, try raising this sexual energy to the third eye and shooting yourself out into the astral to experience the body of light in a sexual context. This is an autoerotic version of the Sleep of Siloam. You can effectively use preliminary ritual activity to prepare for visions in this way.

Connecting with Your Holy Guardian Angel

When you contact your Holy Guardian Angel, you gain access to your essence, your true self, your divine self. There are many ways to approach an autoerotic rite that connects you with your Holy Guardian Angel. This is a highly personal matter and the following is merely one method. In many ways, this sort of autoerotic rite is the ultimate form of masturbation. In it, you masturbate to and for yourself! This does not mean that it's negative or even solipsistic, just that it is extremely personal.

In this method, you will use the ecstatic energies of sex to transcend your normal consciousness and connect with your super-conscious. This sort of work is much more powerful when conducted with your lover, but it is good to start out on your own so that you can fully control the stimulation until you've really mastered your sexual energy.

Start by devoting yourself fully to your Holy Guardian Angel working.[45] Then use your own creativity and inspiration from your Holy Guardian Angel itself to construct the correct pathway to this experience. Adding sexual stimulation changes your state of consciousness in a very unique way, and connects you fairly easily to higher states of consciousness. I actually began my own Holy Guardian Angel work with an exercise very similar to the following.

In order to conduct this exercise, you will most likely need to switch back and forth between arousing and erotic thoughts and more spiritual visualizations. This is perfectly acceptable, as long as you maintain your central focus on establishing contact with the spiritual, using erotic imagery as a catalyst to drive your consciousness toward the ecstasy of union with your Holy Guardian Angel. You can use this exercise to obtain inspiration, illumination, and information from your Holy Guardian Angel whenever you need it.

Invoking Your Holy Guardian Angel Autoerotically

1. Enter a magick trance.
2. Perform whatever opening ritual elements you like, including purification, consecration, oaths, or ceremonial invocations.
3. Sit or lie down, and relax your body and mind fully.
4. When you are in a relaxed and concentrated state, begin to stimulate yourself sexually until you are fully aroused.
5. Maintaining this arousal, visualize your aura, or spiritual body, as a large black egg that surrounds you and is one or two feet taller than you. All around you is darkness.
6. Look up into this darkness and visualize a point of brilliant white light high above you, shining down on your auric egg. This point of light marks the descent of your connection with cosmic consciousness, the descent of your Holy Guardian Angel.
7. Become aware of your desire to experience union with this distant light. This desire stimulates you sexually and arouses the sexual energy in your organs and perineum.
8. Breathe this feeling of desire slowly up through your body, feeling the sexual sensation as it moves up your back, through your sex organs, into your belly. Bring yourself to a near climax, and then draw this energy up to your belly.
9. At the same time, visualize that the point of light above you is growing larger, into a globe, and moving slowly down toward you.
10. Continue feeling your desire for this light, moving it up into your chest. Again you may wish to do this with a near climax.
11. See the light getting larger, continuing to move down toward the top of your head.

12. Continue stimulating yourself, moving the energy up to your neck and throat.

13. As the globe of light gets larger and closer, visualize a beam or ray of light shining down into your black auric egg, down onto the top of your head, turning your auric egg gray. Feel the soft light around you, purifying you within and without.

14. Move your sexual energy, your desire for union with the light, up into your face and your forehead. Feel your desire all through your body mingling with the feelings of purity from the light, and transforming into euphoric bliss.

15. Let the globe of light enter the egg of your aura and touch your head. Visualize and feel an ecstatic influx of brilliant white light filling your whole body and your auric egg.

16. Become totally enveloped in this light. Yield to it. Let it flow pleasurably through you, and let yourself flow into the light. Feel yourself dissolving ecstatically into light. At this point, you can yield to orgasm or not, depending on your personal sense of the correct thing to do at this time. If you do yield to orgasm, be certain that your mind is filled completely with this light as you climax. At first, it may be best not to climax. Instead, fill yourself and dissolve more and more with each near climax, never yielding fully to physical release. You may find yourself completely dissolved into ecstasy.

17. Prolong the experience for as long as you like, returning to normal consciousness and performing closing rituals whenever you are ready.

18. If you have climaxed, consider any fluids produced to be the dew of your Holy Guardian Angel, and consume them ceremoniously.

19. Record your results in your journal.

Practice makes perfect. Regular use of these techniques will make you a master of your sexual energy, and a master of sex. Practice these techniques for quite some time before you begin to use any of them with a partner, because the added stimulation of your partner will make it much harder to control the energies. By practicing these exercises, you will eventually control your orgasmic energies enough to be completely in command of your sexual power. Once you have thoroughly mastered these techniques, you will be ready to move on to practical sex magick.

CHAPTER 5

Sexual Technique and Enhancement

Wisdom says: be strong! Then canst thou bear more joy. Be not animal; refine thy rapture!

—*Liber AL vel Legis, II, 70*

I just made love to the most beautiful woman in the world. In our passion, we were one being—the very essence of the universe itself. I do not know what time passed. I am no longer aware of time at all. I look out upon the world and see paradise. I dwell in the supernal Eden. My lover is truly the divine Sophia, and I the very Logos. If every part of me were to disintegrate into dust at this moment, nothing important would be lost, for what just happened is all that will ever matter, and all that will ever be.

This is the essence of the sacrament of sex. Before turning your sex into a practical operation of magick, turn it into a sacred connection between you and your lover. Let your sex be loving and intimate, truly joining you and your partner on all levels.

Loving Relationships

Love is the key that opens all the treasure houses of heaven and Earth—and hell. There is no power that can destroy love, because it is the whole of universal energy. To experience truly intimate and ecstatic sex within a meaningful relationship that is built on trust and mutual adoration is the essence of love. Love is truly the greatest thing in the universe. To experience love, whether Earthly or spiritual, is to experience the highest and most wonderful thing that can ever be. When you experience love, nothing can harm you. Love given freely is the greatest gift, because you receive it back automatically, through your own feelings of love. If you offer love and it is refused, you still have it.

It is hard to contemplate simply giving love for its own sake without the hope of receiving love back. But it is in doing just this—loving yourself and the beings around you unconditionally—that offers all the healing you could ever need, and brings you to the greatest heights of ecstasy and true joy. When you become free from the fear of loss and give yourself completely to love, when you open your heart, all of life becomes the very image of love. This sort of love is the essence of true courage.

Sexual love is sometimes considered lower than pure spiritual love, but this is totally ridiculous. All love is love, and the courage to love a human being despite all of their faults, treacheries, and limitations, truly seeing the God within—there can be nothing nobler. There are lesser loves that cause nothing but pain, but real love is eternal and imperishable. It is unique to humans among all animals. It is this aspect of your self that is clearly most closely related to God. This is the true power of the Gnostic Sophia within each of us.

We all want love. It is universal. Even the most disturbed and angry person longs to be loved at some level of being. By loving even the mean and awful people in the world, you can heal everything—yourself, your hurt, their hurt. Love is boundless, endless, and harmless, and yet more powerful than any weapon, more powerful than nations, more powerful than life or death.

If you have ever truly loved and lost that love—whether through death or some mistake, or by taking things for granted—then you know true pain. There is no greater pain than lack of love. Yet, having experienced this ultimate pain, you have nothing to fear. For when you have experienced both the joy and pain of love, all other things are as nothing to you. The willingness to risk experiencing this pain is essential to truly loving relationships. "Those who avoid Pain physical or mental remain little Men, and there is no Virtue in them."[46]

Enhanced Relationships

When you are in love, within an intimate and loving relationship, it is a fairly simple matter to enhance the physical pleasure of your sex life. The key is open and honest communication. You need to communicate your sexual needs to your partner in such a way that they can be fulfilled; and in return, you need to listen to your sexual partner's needs. Then you must fulfill them to the best of your ability. If you are hesitant to communicate your own needs or your partner does not share his or her needs, there is really a fundamental problem of trust between you. And where there is a lack of trust, there cannot be true intimacy. In these situations, sex will, at best, be just going through the motions.

Within long-term relationships, some people seem to feel that the sexual fire diminishes. A friend once told me that he really lost interest in having sex with the same woman after three or four sexual connections. After that, it was just boring to him. I found this statement quite sad. He was obviously incapable of establishing any kind of true intimacy with his sex partners, and was basically masturbating in their vaginal cavities. Since his connections were devoid of real love, his love-making was completely empty.

I believe, on the contrary, that the first few times you have sex with a person really just amount to a trial run. Only when you begin to fully understand each other's unique erogenous zones and idiosyncratic turn-ons can sex become really satisfying. Even if you connect instantly with a lover and have amazing initial sex, that sex will grow more wonderful and magical each time, as you grow closer, relate more and more intimately, and learn more and new ways to turn each other on. When you connect fully with your partner, fulfilling his or her needs as yours are fulfilled, sex is always ecstatic and wonderful.

Divine Sex

Once you have established a real sexual intimacy with your partner, turning great sex into divine sex is easy. It is only a matter of recognizing the inherent divinity within your lover, and feeling the loving caresses as a sacred connection. Louis Culling suggests doing this by remaining silent during sex, thereby rendering the act anonymous and focusing completely on a mystical ideal. In this way, he claims, you can turn your sexual partner into a sort of divine sexual surrogate. This is a terribly limiting concept. It neither honors your partner, nor enhances your loving relationship with your partner. Instead, I suggest that you attempt to see the divine that is already intrinsic within your partner, and worship him or her as an inherently sacred avatar of God. See your partner *as* divine, not as some object to personify your fantasy of divinity. There is a Sanskrit term, *namaste* (nah-mah-stay), that is repeated at the beginning and end of all yoga classes. It translates to something approximating, "I honor that place in you in which we are one and the entire Universe dwells." This is the essence of divine sex. See that your partner is divine, and that you are divine, and that your union is a completion of a beautiful sacred polarity.

To Tell or Not to Tell

Some people refrain from telling their sexual partners that they are engaging in sexual magick, or even from sharing the sexual mysticism described above. This is an especially sensitive issue when you are having sex with someone who is not particularly interested in magick. I generally think that it makes for a much more loving and healthy approach if you do include your lover in your work. How can your sex magick be an act of love if one half of the equation is concealing things from the other? It is really best to work with partners who are at least open to your sexual sorcery. If your lover does not know what you are doing, and so is not really including all of his or her energy, why not just work autoerotically?

On the other hand, there is inherent power in the sexual connection, whether both parties are aware of the magick or not, and I have engaged in many highly successful sex-magick operations when my partner was completely unaware of what I was doing. In fact, if you are trying to manifest something, the doubts and negative thoughts of an unbelieving partner may damage the operation. Communication and real intimacy can be lost, however, if you do not share yourself completely. This can degrade your connection with your partner over time, and degrade the effectiveness of your magick as well. If possible, you should tell your partner what you are up to, even if he or she is not particularly interested in occultism. Perhaps you can make a convert!

If you are working with another magician, you should certainly be working together toward the same object, rather than individually willing different things through sex magic. Working at cross-purposes can degrade both efforts. If you want to keep your purposes secret, make arrangements with your partner to "give him- or herself to you." You can then arrange to give yourself to your partner sometime in the future. Of course, there will have to be enough trust in your relationship for this to work well.

Monogamy vs. Polyamory

Every relationship is an opportunity to learn and to grow, to shed what isn't working in your interpersonal skills, and to learn about yourself and the world around you from your partner. This is the alchemy of relationship. By exposing yourself to intimacy and connection, you can discover many of your limitations, fears, and problems, as well as your strengths within a relatively safe situation. You are empowered to cast off your old ways, and awaken to greater heights of consciousness and love. There are, of course, always dangers. You may become obsessed with your partner, or fears and insecurities may tangle you up in negative places. But relationship itself is one of the most powerful learning tools you have at your disposal.

All relationships hold a mysterious power to become more than the sum of their parts. Both partners can be empowered to be and do more than either could be or do alone. Because of this "multiplier effect," many modern sex magicians seem to prefer having multiple sexual partners, rather than focusing on one intimate relationship. The practice of *polyamory* is common in Tantric philosophy, as well as in many Western magical systems. In most of these practices, polyamory occurs within a magical rite, with the new lover acting as a projection screen for the divine. As I said before, this strips away intimacy and, while it may have a powerful temporary effect, does not lead to stable and sustainable growth for either party.

Crowley strongly encouraged polyamory, and practiced it throughout his life. Of course, Crowley never had stable romantic relationships, and never seemed very happy in love for very long at all. When he was in love, the idea of long-term relationship suddenly seemed more appealing. In *Liber Aleph*, when Crowley clearly happens to be in love, he writes: "So also it may be in love, that two souls, meeting, discover each in the other such wealth and richness of light and love, and in one phase of life (or incarnation) or even in many, they exhaust not that treasure."[47] But generally, Crowley advocates taking as many lovers as you want as often as you want, and places no great importance on relationship.

Many other magicians encourage polyamory as a sexual ideal, and view monogamy as a hindrance to full sexual freedom. Indeed, monogamy can be limiting if it is based on fear rather than love and intimacy. If you are staying with a single lover because you fear that no one else will want you, or that you can't do any better, this is no way to build a harmonious love. Polyamory is a great temptation in this sort of relationship, because your needs are not really being fully met by your primary partner.

Polyamory has many flaws, however. I have only seen it work for short periods of time, usually ending in destruction of one or all of the relationships. Most polyamorous relationships start with a couple that invites secondary lovers into their sex life. But who wants to be a secondary lover? The new lovers always seem to vie for a more prominent role and frequently get it, destroying the original relationship in the process. Love triangles or love squares are, by their nature, inherently unstable, and two of the lovers are almost certain to become more attached. In this situation, intimacy is irreparably lost, because everyone is operating out of fear. Most often, all of the lovers end up going their separate ways—frequently with more pain, baggage, and self-doubt than when they started.

Many people engage in polyamory either because their partner is threatening to leave if they do not, or because they need to sleep with a lot of different people in order to feel that they are worthy. Both of these are symptoms of pathological low self-esteem; neither will get you very far. Other people engage in polyamory because they wish to impress others with their prowess and powers of seduction. This can be just another dangerous ego trap.

On the other hand, sex with someone new can be very exciting, and this can have a positive effect on the energies of your magick. I certainly wouldn't say that polyamory is inadvisable, or that it is wrong, but I have never seen it work positively for any length of time. The only times that I have ever seen it work is when none of the participants are particularly attached to each other. But this is a rather empty way of experiencing sexuality and love. Establishing true intimacy with a partner with whom you can really build a life seems a much healthier pursuit. Together you can create deeply ecstatic and loving divine sex—and a harmonious life together at the same time. If your current partner is not someone you'd want to be with for the rest of your life and you are constantly looking at other people lustfully, perhaps you should simply end your current relationship and find a more suitable mate.

Jealousy, Anger, and Possessiveness

Everyone has been hurt badly at some point in life—perhaps many times—and these wounds leave us diminished. But when you try to repair that damage with a relationship, or money, or sex, or food, it simply doesn't work. Only love can fill the void left by emotional wounds. It is the love that you give that heals, not the love you receive. It is a terrible mistake to try to build up your self-worth based on how your partner feels about you, because this forces you to sacrifice your own needs to feed your partner's desires. This leads to jealousy and possessiveness. All of these things take you away from a loving connection entirely.

Instead, love yourself and from this place of personal power, extend your love to someone you find really worthwhile. Your love for your partner must be grounded in your belief that he or she is wonderful, not because he or she is willing to put up with you.

There are things that we all secretly think are terrible about ourselves. Accept these things, or work on changing them, so that you may truly love yourself. Relationships should be based on mutual attraction and feelings of loving compatibility, not on fear.

Most men's sexual urges contain at least some small element of violence. "I'd like to fuck the shit out of her," is not a loving statement, and I've heard similar statements coming out of the lips of far too many men. If anger mingles with your sexual urges, however, you will not desire to experience the bliss of union, but instead will just be scratching an itch—and perhaps an angry itch at that. Sexuality must be a loving connection between two people or it is merely masturbation with a partner, or perhaps even something unhealthy. If you wish to enhance your deep sexual connection with your lover, you must remove anger and violence from your way of thinking about sex. You can, of course, be wild and animalistic, groping and tearing at each other. Just make sure that your passionate "violence" is grounded in love.

Group Sex

Like polyamorous relationships, group sex seems like a dangerous and unstable dead-end to this particular sexual sorcerer. While I have engaged in a few pretty sexy orgies, I have never been involved with group sex magick that resembled anything even approximating useful magick. The sexual energy tends to be diffuse, unorganized, and directed (if it is directed at all) more at the smutty pleasure of debauchery than at anything transformative, transcendent, or evolutionary. Most participants seem more interested in "getting off" than anything at all magical or even loving. I admit, however, that this may be the result of my own limitations, or the limitations of the people with whom I've surrounded myself.

I have seen a great deal more harm than good come out of group sex in a magical context. I once attended an invocatory group ritual that descended into an orgiastic sex frenzy focused on one woman who had taken on an invocation of Astarte after consuming a capsule of ecstasy. She ended up having wild sex with at least five partners (none of whom was me). I felt very uncomfortable, knowing that she was going to regret this later, and left the temple before it all ended.

If you are interested in exploring group sex magick, please arrange things carefully in advance and make sure that all participants are really aware of what is going on. I still doubt that there is much utility in this sort of work in today's social context. Such events too closely resemble mere "swinger" orgy situations, and their energy always seems dark and ugly, rather than divine. But then, I have explored the matter to my own satisfaction. Perhaps you need to explore these things as well, in order to discover your own True Will in this matter. I do really strongly feel, however, that you gain more from intimate one-on-one encounters.

How to Be a Great Lover

I have not always been a very good lover. I used to be sexually selfish, incapable of controlling my orgasmic release, and often inconsiderate. But I have learned to be delighted sexually by giving pleasure to my partner as well as receiving it. As I gained greater control of my own physical sexual responses, it transformed my whole experience of sexuality. I learned to listen to women's desires, and to take great pleasure in fulfilling them. I strongly believe that my desire for true intimacy and my love for giving pleasure have made me a much better lover—and my partners seem to agree.

In preparing this manuscript, I interviewed a wide range of women, nearly all of whom took a fairly dim view of the majority of their past male lovers. Gentlemen, you do not rate very highly! It seems that men in general are rude and selfish lovers who finish far too quickly. If you finish with your sexual experience before your partner has even one orgasm, you are hardly a sexual sorcerer, my friend. Unless, of course, your partner does not want to have an orgasm for some specific reason. If sex is just about your own pleasure, you are failing to honor your partner, the feminine divine, or even your own anima.

Here are a few tips that can help men become better lovers:

- Be clean, and not smelly.
- Go slowly. Start slowly and continue more slowly than you think is necessary. Then go even more slowly. Never be rough or brutal, unless your partner is specifically turned on by roughness.
- Do not focus all of your attention on either yours or your partner's genitalia. Worship the whole body. Surely there are other parts of your partner's anatomy that you find enticing. Erotically and worshipfully stimulate your partner's whole body.
- Observe what stimulates your partner, continue doing these things, and expand on them.
- When playing with or orally stimulating the clitoris, do this for her pleasure and also yours. Do not behave as if you are just trying to moisten her vagina enough to stick your penis in. Enjoy her labia and clitoris for its own sake. Worship her genitals as the embodiment of the sacred female energy.
- Do not over-stimulate the clitoris, as it is extremely sensitive. It may be better to stimulate the area around the clitoris primarily. Would you want a giant tongue repeatedly licking the head of your penis?
- Do not penetrate the vagina until it is really ready to be penetrated. If it's hard to get your penis in, this almost invariably means that you are hurting your partner. She may not tell you, because she doesn't want to embarrass you or ruin the mood. Just don't stick it in until her vagina is very wet and open for your penis.
- Take the time to arouse your partner fully with words, kissing, and touching. Worship her.
- Listen to your partner when she tells you what she wants sexually, and do it. Ask her what she likes if she's not telling you. If she won't tell you, then she doesn't feel entirely comfortable with her sexuality or with you. Make her comfortable by being kind and loving in all of your relationship.

Women also need to become more considerate and affectionate lovers. Try some of the following ideas to help you to become a more proficient lover:

- Communicate what you want in a sexy and enticing way. Seduce your partner with your desires so that he wants to fulfill them.
- Don't criticize your partner's performance in any way. Instead, try to come up with positive and erotic ways to get your needs fulfilled.
- Put his penis in your mouth, and like it. He will. Don't treat it like a labor or a chore in order to get him to go down on you. Treat it as a worshipful act, to arouse the sacred male energy. Worship his penis.
- Let him know how much you love his penis. Admire it as your favorite penis ever, both verbally and with your actions.
- Don't neglect other parts of his body. Although some men may think they are only interested in their penis, all men secretly like to be adored in many other places as well. Men are sometimes very shy about communicating this sort of information, so don't be afraid to explore.
- Say sexy things to your partner while he adores you. Tell him how much he turns you on (unless he specifically doesn't like this).
- Don't ever pretend to have an orgasm. This will create distance rather than connection between you. If you are not interested in continuing with the sex act, just lovingly say that you want to stop for now. If he does not like it, he is not a very nice gentleman.

To really understand more about your partner's needs, try some of the following simple techniques:

Sexual discussion: Find a time when you can have an intimate conversation with your lover—an exchange in which both of you feel comfortable and loving. Do not try to have this sort of conversation right after sex, or after an argument. Ask questions like these, and try to make them fun and sexy: What turns you on? Which parts of your body do you wish I touched more? What have I (or past lovers) done that you don't like? Which sexual positions do you prefer? What sexual fantasies can we fulfill together? Try to really understand as much as you can about your partner's needs and desires. When you are finished, try fulfilling some of these desires right away. Remember to write down your partner's needs in your journal, so that you can satisfy them as completely as possible from now on.

Mutual masturbation: One of the best ways to understand how to please your partner sexually is to watch him or her masturbate. This can also be incredibly arousing for you. Set aside some time to watch each other masturbate individually. Notice how your partner touches him or herself, the kinds of pressure, the places, etc. When you feel as if you know what your partner is doing, try masturbating each other. Feel free to use both hands and mouth. Enjoy giving your partner pleasure. Don't forget to write down your observations and experiences later, so that you can reference them in the future.

Sex magick discussion: Have a real discussion about how sex magick can be a part of your relationship. Conduct this conversation lovingly, at a time when you both feel open to it. Don't ever put any pressure on your partner. In this conversation, you may discover that your needs and desires concerning sexual magick are quite different from your partner's. Compromise may be necessary. Be careful not to insult your partner's sexual abilities in this discussion. Questions like: "Can you really hold out for a half hour or more?" will cause pain, not a greater understanding of each other. If one partner lies or attempts to placate the other with offers that will not be fulfilled, there is no point to this conversation. If you are not presently in a relationship, simply take some time to think about your own goals and desires with sexual magick. Always record your thoughts and feelings in your journal.

Magical chastity—third type: For at least a month, and preferably on a permanent basis, completely dedicate your sexuality to magick. If you are in a relationship, be sure to have the discussion described above. If you are single, you do not need to have a specific magical goal connected to all of your sexual expression. Instead, simply be aware at all times that your sexual thoughts, feelings, and encounters are magical, and devote yourself to seeing the divine and magical nature of your sexuality. Record your experiences in your journal.

Sex for the divine lover: Make your lovers avatars of the god or goddess of love and sex. Worship them. Have sex with them completely for them, fulfilling all their needs and not being concerned about your own at all. Do not even bother to have an orgasm, unless your partners specifically tell you it will increase their pleasure for you to climax. Record your experiences in your journal.

Sex with the divine lover: See your lover as the embodiment of holiness; make love seeking to connect to all that is divine within your partner. Let your lovemaking be ecstatic and passionate; seek to unite yourself with the divine through your love. Record your experiences in your journal.

Sex and Your Holy Guardian Angel

Sex-magical operations can bring you dangerously close to using your sexual partner as a mere masturbation tool if they are not conducted with a spirit of love. But they can bring about a beautiful true connection if both partners participate, seeking the divine together through the passion of love. You connect to the universal through your partner—it is as much a part of your lover as it is of yourself. Your partner is a divine being, and your love for him or her a divine love. Your Holy Guardian Angel is reflected in the eyes of your beloved. Through this love, you are empowered to be and do more than would otherwise be possible. Sometimes, through a chance word or phrase, your lover will speak to you directly with the voice of the divine. You have but to listen. Your love for your partner is the flame that awakens your connection to your own divinity.

The following exercise is essentially the same as the one for invoking Your Holy Guardian Angel autoerotically (pages 124–125), except you will now conduct it with a lover. This very simple and beautiful experience works best if both partners perform the exercise at the same time, though this certainly is not necessary. It may also be useful to experiment with one partner conducting, and the other facilitating, the experience. Again, I offer just one way of approaching this here. Your creativity will supply you with infinite variations.

Invoking Your Holy Guardian Angel with a Partner

1. Enter a magick trance with your partner, and perform whatever opening ritual elements you prefer, including purification, consecration, oaths, or ceremonial invocations.
2. For the moment, forget about the working and simply arouse each other lovingly for as long as you like, and then begin to make love.
3. Once you are blissfully intermingled, begin to visualize your aura, or spiritual body, as a large black egg that is one or two feet taller and wider than you. Both you and your lover are encompassed in this egg. All around you is darkness.
4. Visualize the point of brilliant white light—the essence of your connection with cosmic consciousness, the descent of your Holy Guardian Angel—as hidden deep within your lover.
5. Become aware of your desire to experience union with this distant light within your lover. Let this desire bring you to the edge of climax, pulling back at the point of no return, and drawing the ecstasy through your sex organs into your belly.
6. At the same time, visualize the point of light within your lover growing into a globe of pure white light, and coming closer to you.
7. Continue feeling your desire for this light as you near orgasm. Draw the ecstasy into your chest and see the light deep within your lover getting larger, brighter, closer.
8. Bring yourself to near-climax again, moving the energy up to your neck and throat. See the globe of light within your lover continuing to grow larger and closer.
9. Visualize a ray of light shining out into your black auric egg from within your lover, turning your auric egg gray. Feel the soft light around you, purifying you within and without.
10. As you approach another climax, move your sexual energy, your desire for union with the light, up into your face and your forehead. Feel your desire all through your body mingling with the feelings of purity from the light—a euphoric bliss.
11. Let the globe of light emerge through the heart of your love. Visualize and feel an ecstatic influx of brilliant white light filling your whole body and your auric egg.
12. Become totally enveloped in this light. Yield to it, letting it flow pleasurably through you. Let yourself flow into the light and into your partner. Feel yourself dissolving ecstatically into light. At this

point, you may yield to orgasm or not, depending on your personal sense of the correct thing to do at this time. If you do yield to orgasm, be certain that your mind is filled completely with this light as you climax. At first, it may be best not to climax, instead, filling yourself and dissolving more and more with each near-climax, never yielding fully to physical release. In doing this, you may find yourself completely dissolved into ecstasy.

13. Allow yourself to experience whatever you experience for as long as you like. Return to normal consciousness whenever you feel the need. If you have climaxed, consider any fluids produced to be the dew of your Holy Guardian Angel, and consume them ceremoniously—preferably with your partner. Perform any closing rituals you desire whenever you are ready.

14. Record your results in your journal.

Sexual Bornless One

This rite may seem overly complex to some, but it is essentially the same technique Crowley used to connect with his Holy Guardian Angel. To perform it, you must merge your sexual experience with your experience of the body of light—your active imagination—conducting the ritual elements in an astral temple. Your sexual partner becomes the avatar of elemental beings, as well as your Holy Guardian Angel. You alternate your focus between the physical and spiritual sensations that flow throughout the experience. The "inner temple" of *The New Hermetics* provides a simple way to approaching this, though your own astral temple may be as elaborate as you like.[48]

This technique contains strings of "barbarous words" that date back two thousand years. These magical words of power derive from the Hellenistic Hermetic formulae of ancient Alexandria. Many people find these words quite powerful and inspiring, but you can also simply perform the visualizations, omitting the words, as they require a large amount of memorization. I've adapted the invocations to more modern language, but you can use the originals if you prefer. This rite itself is similar in structure to the Lesser Ritual of the Pentagram, though you conduct the ritual elements solely in your active imagination, not by physically moving around a temple. You may astrally trace invoking pentagrams of the appropriate elements if you wish, but I have left them out of the instructions for simplicity's sake.

Invoking the Bornless One

1. Enter a magick trance with your partner, and perform whatever opening ritual elements you prefer—purification, consecration, oaths, or ceremonial invocations.
2. For the moment, forget about the working and simply arouse each other lovingly for as long as you like, and then begin to make love.
3. Once you begin having sex, imagine yourself within an astral temple, surrounded by the four elements; air to the east (in front of you), fire to the south (on your right), water to the west (behind you), and earth to the north (on your left).
4. Visualize a shining globe of white brilliance above your head. Allow it to become larger and brighter. Feel the light of your Holy Guardian Angel glowing above you, in your astral temple, and, at the same time, within your partner. Feel this light entering you through the ecstatic connection with your partner. Say to yourself silently, or with your partner:

I invoke you Bornless One, beingness that has no beginning and no end.

You who create the Earth and the heavens.

You who create the night and the day.

You who create the darkness and the light.

You are myself made perfect that no one has ever seen.

You are matter, destroying to create, you are force, destroying to create.

You have distinguished the just and the unjust, the female and the male.

You produce the seed and the fruit, making all to love and to hate one another.

You create the moist and the dry and that which nourishes all life.

I am your prophet to whom you have given your mysteries.

Hear me, for I am yours. You are myself made perfect.

5. Now look to the east of your temple and see billowing clouds of yellowish air before you. See a giant golden–yellow being forming in the billows of cloud. This is the guardian of the element air. At the same time, see this being as your lover, and your lover as this being. As you make love, feel yourself becoming one with your partner and this being, growing and expanding into an airy being of power. Feel the awesome elemental power of air within you, glowing brightly. As you near orgasm, draw the energy back through you and project it into your partner. Allow yourself to expand, filling the universe more and more with each word, as you say to yourself the sacred words:

AR . . . THI-A-O . . . RHE-I-BET . . . A-THE-LE-BER-SET . . . A . . . BE-LA-THA . . . AB-E-U . . . EB-E-U . . . PHI . . . THE-TA-SO-E . . . IB . . . THI-A-O

6. Expand into an infinite airy being and say:

Hear my word and make all spirits subject to my command, so that every spirit, whether of the heavens or of the air, of the earth or beneath the earth, on land or in the water, and every force, feeling and form in the cosmos is mine to command.

7. Look to your right and see flames and a giant fiery-red being forming in them. This is your guardian of the element fire. At the same time, see this being as your lover, and your lover as this being. As you make love, feel yourself becoming one with your partner and this being, growing and expanding into a fiery being of power. As you near orgasm, draw the energy back through you and project it into your partner. Allow yourself to expand, filling the universe more and more with each word, as you say to yourself the sacred words:

AR-O-GO-GO-RU-BRA-O . . . SO-TO-U . . . MU-DO-RI-O . . . PHA-LAR-TA-O . . . O-O-O . . . A-PE

8. Expand into an infinite fiery being and say:

Hear my word and make all spirits subject to my command, so that every spirit, whether of the heavens or of the air, of the earth or beneath the earth, on land or in the water, and every force, feeling and form in the cosmos is mine to command.

9. Visualize undulating waves of water behind you, and a giant pulsing blue being forming in the flow of water. This is the guardian of the element water. At the same time, see this being as your lover, and your lover as this being. As you make love, feel yourself becoming one with your partner and this being, growing and expanding into a watery being of power. As you near orgasm, draw the energy back through you and project it into your partner. Allow yourself to expand, filling the universe more and more with each word, as you say to yourself the sacred words:

*RU-A-BRA-I-A-O . . . MRI-O-DOM . . . BA-BA-LON-
BAL-BIN-A-BAFT . . . A-SAL-ON-A-I . . . A-PHE-NI-A-O
. . . I . . . PHO-TETH . . . A-BRA-SAX . . . A-E-O-O-U . . .
I-SCHU-RE*

10. Expand into an infinite watery being and say:

*Hear my word and make all spirits subject to my command, so that
every spirit, whether of the heavens or of the air, of the earth or
beneath the earth, on land or in the water, and every force, feeling
and form in the cosmos is mine to command.*

11. Visualize rocky structures forming on your left and a giant earthy black being forming among the structures. This is the guardian of the element earth. At the same time, see this being as your lover, and your lover as this being. As you make love, feel yourself becoming one with your partner and this being, growing and expanding into an earthy being of power. As you near orgasm, draw the energy back through you and project it into your partner. Allow yourself to expand, filling the universe with each word, as you say to yourself the sacred words:

*MA . . . BAR-RI-O . . . I-O-EL . . . KO-THA . . . A-THO-
RE-BA-LO . . . A-BRA-OT*

12. Expand into an infinite earthy being and say:

*Hear my word and make all spirits subject to my command, so that
every spirit, whether of the heavens or of the air, of the earth or
beneath the earth, on land or in the water, and every force, feeling
and form in the cosmos is mine to command.*

13. Become aware of the shining globe of white brilliance above your head and within your partner. Allow this to become larger and brighter, filling you with light. As you near orgasm, draw the energy back through you and project it into your partner. Allow yourself to flow into the light and your lover as the light flows into you. Dissolve into the light of your Holy Guardian Angel as you say the sacred words:

A-OT . . . A-BA-OT . . . BA-SA-U-M . . . I-SAK . . . SA-BA-O . . . I-A-O

This is the ruler of the universe who the winds fear. This is who made voice and all things were created. Ruler, master, helper.

I-E-O-U . . . PUR . . . I-O-U . . . PUR . . . I-A-OTH . . . I-A-E-O . . . I-O-O-U . . . A-BRA-SAX . . . SA-BRI-AM . . . O-O . . . U-U . . . E-U . . . O-O.. U-U . . . A-DO-NA-I . . . E-DE . . . E-DU . . . AN-GE-LO-STON-THE-ON . . . AN-LA-LA . . . LA-I . . . GA-I-A . . . A-E-PE . . . DI-A-THAR-NA . . . THO-RON

I am the Bornless One

Having sight in the feet: strong and the immortal fire

I am the truth

I am the one in lightning and in thunder

My sweat is the rain that showers the earth with life

My mouth is ever flaming

I am the maker and begetter of the light!

I am the grace of the world.

The heart girt with a serpent is my name

I-A-O . . . SA-BA-O

14. At any time during this final invocation, you may yield to orgasm or not, depending on your inclination and the circumstances.
15. Cease being anything and allow yourself to be with infinity.
16. Allow yourself to experience whatever you experience for as long as you like. Return to normal consciousness whenever you feel the need. If you have climaxed, consider any fluids produced

to be the dew of your Holy Guardian Angel, and consume them ceremoniously, preferably with your partner. Perform any closing rituals you like whenever you are ready.

17. Record your results in your journal.

Aleister Crowley's Star Sapphire ritual[49] can be adapted as a sexual rite in essentially the same way. In the state of ecstasy produced by either rite, try to sense what it is you want to do with your life. This is an excellent time to consider your True Will, as you will be in an extremely exalted state. You can use many different creative ways to explore your True Will: draw pictures, write poems, or simply let yourself unfold to yourself. As you come to realizations about your own nature, discuss these thoughts and your secret dreams with your partner. What does your lover think of your thoughts? What are your lover's secret dreams about life and the future? Record everything in your journal.

CHAPTER 6

Practical Sex Magick

Also the mantras and spells; the obeah and the wanga; the work of the wand and the work of the sword; these he shall learn and teach.

—*Liber AL vel Legis, I, 37*

Now, we move to the practicalities of the miracle of sex magick itself. The great thing about sex magick is that it is extremely powerful, while at the same time incredibly portable. You do not need an elaborate temple or wands or ceremonies or anything other than your genitals. So, although you have learned a number of rituals here, you may rarely use them in your practical work. Sex magick must, first and foremost, be sexy, and watching your partner trace pentagrams in the air may not be the sexiest thing in the world. Or maybe it is! If that's your turn-on, so be it.

The power of sex magick is not overrated. It is truly one of the most amazing phenomena; you will be amazed again and again by how effective this simple method of conducting magick can be. Many writers create elaborate rituals and extended operations that involve multiple sex acts and offer them as ways to help your work. But this is really unnecessary. Sex magick is simple and efficacious. One decisive fiat[50] is often enough to accomplish your desire. In Crowley's sex-magical record, *Rex de Arte Regia,*[51] he frequently conducts more than one sexual operation in a day. The frequency and spontaneity with which these acts occur seem to indicate that he used no elaborate ceremonies whatsoever, at most performing some sort of ritual activity in his "body of light."

Many magicians use mental rituals, performing elements of ceremony silently in their "bodies of light," while their physical selves continue with sexual relations. The Bornless One exercise from the last chapter is an example of this technique. This may or may not work for you. As long as your intentions are clear and you are able to direct your own inner energies and connect with the energies of your partner, you can conduct sex-magick operations with no ceremonial or ritualistic elements at all.

Though ceremonial invocation is not always necessary, it can sometimes play a critical role in creating a real connection to the divine through sex. It is this divine connection that forges the crucial link between sexuality and magick. I once conducted a ceremony with a sex-magical lover in which we intentionally used no sex at all, only ritual. However, once we had invoked our gods, Hades and Kore, we were both struck with an irresistible passion and enjoyed one of the most beautiful experiences of mystical sex that either of us had ever had.

In the exercises that follow, I reference ceremonial elements, but these are optional. Feel free to omit them at will. As you start out with sex magick, however, it is probably wise to use more ceremony, rather than less. Although ceremonial aspects are not absolutely essential, they may help you create the proper atmosphere for magick. Once you are more experienced and have dedicated your sexual energy to magick over a period of time, your sex-magical experiences can and will be more and more organic.

I must admit that there have been several occasions on which I found myself engaged in a spontaneous sexual encounter not dedicated to a specific purpose. On those occasions, I formulated a purpose right in the middle of the sex act. And in cases where the purpose was some sort of manifestation or magical end, I succeeded every time in getting my result. So there are no hard and fast rules. The mysteries of sex magick are beyond rational comprehension.

The Typology of Practical Sex Magick

There are essentially four different kinds of sexual magick that blend into one another in several places. Let's look at them each individually.

THAUMATURGY

Thaumaturgy means, "the making of miracles." This is magick in its most traditional sense. The magician wants something, and so conducts an operation to get it through the divine magical power at his or her disposal. The purpose is to obtain something material or substantial through manipulating the subtle planes.

There are six things that people generally want from magick: health, money, love, power, or revenge, and protection from other people's magick. Interestingly, all of these have a sexual basis concealed beneath the surface. All of these ends can be achieved through sexual thaumaturgy. Because sex is a creative and loving act, it lends itself most readily to creative and loving ends. Though you can direct sex magick destructively, this is not the best use of your energy. Nor is it good or healthy for your loving relationship.

Generally speaking, this form of sex-magical work is conducted in pairs. It is the connection between self and not-self that completes the cosmic circuit and opens you up to your divine miracle-making power. It is the Formula of the Rosy Cross. When working alone, autoerotically, sex magick usually consists of connecting with some spiritual entity, thus making the connection between self and not-self on a subtler plane. These practices are called *theurgy* and *goetia*. In working sexual thaumaturgy with a partner, however, you can also invoke a being or beings from the subtle planes, thereby combining elements of theurgy or goetia into your thaumaturgy.

THEURGY

Theurgy is the science and art of communing with the gods. From a sex-magical perspective, this is any operation whose intent is to invoke archetypal beings, forces, and ideas. This includes a whole range of activities, from invoking specific god forms such as Isis or Dionysus, to simply invoking a quality, as in the Qodosh practices of the G∴B∴G∴ or the Tirauclairism of Paschal Beverly Randolph. In the next chapter, we will explore a number of these sexual invocation techniques and practices.

While sexual thaumaturgy is most often practiced between two people, theurgy is often practiced by a single person autoerotically. Theurgy can easily be conducted by a couple, however, and can even involve the invocation of a divine pair, such as Isis and Osiris, or Mars and Venus, or any other appropriate divine couple. This is the essence of the "Great Rite" of witchcraft.

Theurgy can have multiple purposes. You may wish to invoke some god form or idea to gain transcendental knowledge of the archetype; you may wish to obtain some sort of magical favor; or you may wish to gain some of the power or character of the god to compensate for a deficiency in your own character.

GOETIA

For our purposes, Goetia is the general practice of calling forth spirits. This is evocation, which consists of contacting forces, beings, and intelligences that are somehow less than human—elementals, demons, and atavistic throwbacks to our bestial evolutionary past. Goetia helps you understand and direct these subconscious forces toward your own growth. The practice of sexual interaction with succubae and incubi also fits into this category.

Goetia also includes the creation of artificial elementals and the creation of familiar spirits to accomplish things in much the same way as thaumaturgy. Like theurgy, however, goetic sex magick can be conducted with a partner or autoerotically.

MYSTICISM

While thaumaturgy, theurgy, and goetia all certainly have mystical elements—most particularly the theurgic practices—I mean something specific when I talk about mystical sex. Mystical sex encompasses those sexual encounters specifically directed toward transcending individual consciousness and merging with the divine through union with your lover. In this, there are no symbols or archetypal structures like the Holy Guardian Angel or a god form. Instead, you merge into the silent ocean of the transcendent.

Mystical sex involves more than an energetic raising of your sexual experience directly into higher planes. It entails a shifting of your consciousness into the gap between thoughts and escaping the mundane directly through the ecstasy of sex. All sex-magical operations result in this experience to a certain extent, but we will explore ways to move into this state explicitly in a later chapter.

Essentials of Practical Sex Magick

For those of you who may have skipped right to this section without reading the rest of the book—shame on you! But now that you are here, we'll get right to the heart of the matter. The basic outline of a sex-magick operation can be given in a few simple steps. Over the rest of this book, we will modify this basic structure toward various specific ends. In many cases, however, this simple procedure may be enough by itself to accomplish what you need.

Sex magick is an energetic disturbance on the subtle planes, whose action carries the weight of higher consciousness. From a mythological and metaphysical point of view, spiritual energies accumulate when you have sex with the intention of incarnating a new human being. These energies are intrinsic to all sexual activity—heterosexual, masturbatory, or homosexual. As the sex energies are raised, they alert something on a spiritual level that reproduction is taking place. This happens automatically, just as the sperm cells jet out of the penis automatically, even if a male is wearing a condom or just masturbating. By invoking specific archetypal energies previous to the sex-magick rite, the sexually accumulated spiritual energies will relate to the invoked forces. As you visualize and direct your own sexual energies toward your goal, the accumulating spiritual energies follow your direction. As you connect more and more deeply with your daimon, your Holy Guardian Angel, your super-conscious, you connect more and more deeply with the subtle causal pathways that can bring about your desired result. This is the whole secret of sex magick.

Successful workings take place mostly within the framework of nature's laws, so your magick should always conform to these. In other words, create only that which is conceivable within the realm of possibility; don't chase the impossible or improbable. If you have no job, no friends, no relatives, and are sitting trapped in the desert, it is unlikely that a working to obtain a large sum of money will be very effective. This is a general guideline more than a hard-and-fast rule. Strange things occur from time to time, and miracles do manifest right out of the realm of the impossible. But if you constantly chase the impossible, you will fail often enough that you may give up on sex magick altogether. If you spend your energy manifesting your True Will, you will see the magnitude of this miraculous power!

If both people in a sex act are magicians, and both are actively engaged in the magical working, their object must be singular. Don't both will different or distinct ends, or you will confuse things. At the very least, it will certainly weaken both your efforts. If you are interested in two different things—well, that's just more opportunity for sex!

Some magicians prefer to work with non-magicians for this very reason, so that the working can be singular. However, many people have told me that they do not at all like the idea of being left out when sex magick is going on. So, unless you plan to create distance rather than connection in your relationship, I strongly suggest communicating your intention clearly with all your sexual partners if at all possible.

Try the following simple technique several times, adjusting it as necessary to your own personal requirements. We will discuss talismans, invocations, and sexual Eucharist in more detail later, but you are probably ready to conduct this operation right now if you choose to.

Performing Basic Sex Magick

1. Decide on a specific magical goal. You can make a talisman, or choose a god or spirit to represent this goal. If you are working a spell remotely, obtain something belonging to the absent person as a "magical link," and have it present during the operation. You can also write a mantra or short spell to summarize your intention, and repeat it throughout the sex act.
2. Get into a magical state of mind with your partner. This can be through bathing, meditations, and/or rituals.
3. Invoke the forces congruent with your magical intention, either through ritual or some other means like simple visualization. Be sure to recognize the divine power in yourself and your partner. This may include invocations of the Holy Guardian Angel or daimon.
4. Stimulate each other sexually to full arousal. For the time being, leave aside the purpose of the rite. It will remain in the background of your consciousness if you have properly formulated your intent and correctly invoked appropriate magical energies.
5. Once you and your partner are completely aroused, begin having sex. Make the sex passionate and loving. Focus your thoughts and energies on the purpose of the operation, continuously visualizing that you are preparing to incarnate your force or desire. Your passionate connection with your partner is the path of manifestation for your desire. You can start to use your mantra or spell to keep you focused.
6. Allow the sexual fires to be as ecstatic as possible.
7. If you begin to lose your arousal, change your focus briefly to include just the beauty and seductiveness of your partner to build

up sexual energy. Then, as soon as you regain focus, immediately redirect this energy toward your purpose.

8. Come to the edge of orgasm with your partner several times, then pull the energy inward and upward using one of the energy-movement techniques we discussed. The number of times you do this may correspond to the nature of the operation—for instance, seven for an intention related to planetary force of Venus. Draw this loving ecstasy out as long and as passionately as possible, so that both partners enter the ecstatic realm of the transcendent over and over again.

9. Finally, when you do yield to genital orgasm, do it simultaneously if possible, directing the purpose of the operation into that ecstasy together.

10. Gather the sexual fluids and place them on your talisman or "magical link" if you used one. Consume the rest with your partner as a Eucharist. In eating the fluids, recognize that you are taking the energy of the rite into your bodies as a sacred communion with each other and the divine. In this way, the power of the operation becomes a part of your lives. If the operation is specifically to benefit one operant only, that partner can eat all of the fluids alone.

11. Perform any closing rites, and record your experience in your journal.

Magical Chastity—Final Type

Now that you are going to start actively creating miracles with sex magick, we must come back to the subject of magical chastity. You have now practiced three different types of magical chastity, so there is only one step left. This is to devote all of your energy, both sexual and non-sexual, to discovering your True Will and accomplishing or manifesting it. Work along these lines only with your sexual magick and devote yourself to your True Will at all times. If your work is full of caprice and foolishness it will start to fail more and more and probably bring you to misery. Why are you on this planet? Spend your time answering this question, in thought, action, and deed from now on. Record your thoughts on this matter in your journal.

Practical Considerations

Appropriate incense, music, silken cloths, tapestries or draperies, and colored candles can play a useful role in all of your work, creating an atmosphere of magick and a sensual mood at the same time. Use your own creative imagination, or one of the many books available on this subject, to guide you in your choices. Table 7 gives some general correspondence for planetary and elemental work. I leave the choice of music completely up to you.

Some sexual authorities suggest fasting in preparation for sex magick. While this may or may not be necessary in your work, you should cer-

Table 7. Elemental and Planetary Correspondences

Planet/Element	Color	Incense
Saturn	indigo or black	myrrh
Jupiter	blue or purple	cedar
Mars	red	tobacco (or red pepper or other hot scents)
Sun	yellow/gold	frankincense
Venus	green	benzoin
Mercury	orange	sandalwood
Moon	blue, purple, silver	camphor
fire	red	cinnamon
water	blue or green	cedar
air	blue or yellow	sandalwood
earth	green, yellow, black, or brown	myrrh

tainly not eat a sizeable meal within an hour of any operation so that you are physically able to be fully joyful and flexible in your sex. Tantrics eat a little taboo food before their rites, but certainly not a full meal. You can use wine as a mild intoxicant at the start of your operation, but all stimulants should be used in moderation so as not to impair your focus or your will.

You may wish to consider astrological and seasonal influences during your workings, though I must admit I almost never do. Many magicians swear by this practice, however, and it may be helpful to consider the planetary correspondences of the days of the week when you plan planetary workings (see Table 8). The phases of the Moon can also lend some macrocosmic force to your workings if you confine active, creative, sex-magical work to the waxing Moon.

You may want to perform your rite only once for a specific purpose, as this sends a clear and singular force into the universe. You can also try building a force over time through multiple rites. This should be the result of conscious choice, however, and not by caprice or impatience to obtain your goal. I know a sex magician who performed a weekly Jupiterean sex-magick rite every Thursday for years, and was very happy with his results. Use your own intuition in these matters and experiment until you find what works for you. The most important thing is your passion—for your partner and your work.

Table 8. Planetary Correspondences of the Days of the Week

Monday	Moon
Tuesday	Mars
Wednesday	Mercury
Thursday	Jupiter
Friday	Venus
Saturday	Saturn
Sunday	Sun

The results of sex-magick operations usually appear quickly, often more quickly than through any other form of magick. But don't be disheartened if there is a delay. I have nearly always seen some sort of result, even if it eventually turns out to be disastrous.

Effective Visualization Techniques

There are dozens of ways to visualize the movement of energies and ideas in sexual magick. The following are only my suggestions and, though they have proven very effective for me, you will find your own best ways of doing things as you become a true sexual sorcerer.

The sexual connection is a metaphysical completion of the very essence of yourself. It is important, therefore, that you view your sexual partner as the twin half of your being. If you invoke a god or gods, your partner becomes the chosen consort of this god. Your lover is that special element of your own Holy Guardian Angel that you seek. When you find it, you will finally experience the totality. Your partner is the other half of your little universe. You can understand that which is universal through your connection.

As you begin having sex, focus on your intention, and have your partner focus on it too. This focus can be on a series of images, or just on an abstract idea. Silently chanting a related mantra or rhyming couplet can help. The cycles of pelvic thrusts in your sex may also correspond to the nature of the operation, like knocks or circumambulations.[52] This will connect your focus with your partner as well.

As you near orgasm, depending on your personal level of control, draw the sex energy up through your body, into your head, and above to the white light of super-conscious, imagining the magical intention going along with it. You can either leave the energy there above your head, or draw it down the front of your body and deposit it into your belly cauldron. Either way seems to work. You can also direct the energy into your partner, circulating it between the two of you. At this point, you should allow your partner to experience similar ecstasies. Share in the joy and connection, while maintaining your own concentration on the operation. This can also be done mutually.

After you've done this a few times, you will begin to experience periods of gnosis and/or black-out, in which the sexual ecstasy running through your body simply overwhelms you. When this starts to happen, your must focus your will more clearly, directing your energies toward your goal.

After a half-hour to an hour, allow yourself to climax. With the orgasm, all of the energies you've collected will rush together into the fluids released. I used to think holding out for a half-hour before orgasm was impossible. I know now that it is not only possible; it is wonderful. If you can, reach your climax at the same time as your partner. I also used to think simultaneous orgasm was a myth, but I've since learned that, if both partners are relatively in control of their own orgasmic reflex, this is not nearly as hard as it sounds.

Female orgasm is somewhat different in character than male orgasm, so a woman's exact formula for sex magick is slightly different. The male delivers his semen into the female, but there is no equivalent exchange of fluids into the male, even if the female does ejaculate something. Many female sexual magicians describe their techniques for dealing with the magical energies at orgasm in fairly male terms. They speak of launching their energy out of their vaginas, or their solar plexus, or some other chakra. While this is perfectly reasonable in auto-erotic female workings, in heterosexual sex magick, this really misses the target. If you launch your energy away from your womb, you don't add to the elixir being created there.

Strangely, most of these same women described their actual orgasms in exactly the way I feel the energy should flow within the female during sex magick. The flow of orgasm is up into the body in rolling waves, from the genitals, into the whole torso, and beyond. This flow of energy should be allowed to follow its own path, along with the flow of the male's energetic release, and then crystallize back through the will into the vaginal cavity. The fluid gathered there forms the basis of the elixir.

The Elixirs

Now we must get into sticky territory. (Please forgive the pun. I couldn't resist!) At the end of the thaumaturgic rite, you are left with a small mass of fluid in the vaginal cavity that is the physical manifestation of all of the energies you built up with your working. Traditionally, sex magicians collect this substance by sucking it out, and then eat it. This substance is the very body of your will—it is your magical child, the little god of will you've incarnated magically.

This should be considered a very holy substance—the Eucharist of sex magick. It is the elixir of life, according to Crowley. But most people find the idea of eating this sexual residue rather repulsive. Be honest. You probably do too. Some people really like to eat it; most people do not. But if you are going to be a sexual sorcerer, you are going to have to get past any squeamish feelings about the bodily fluids of sex. And if you are going to be a truly powerful sorcerer, you are going to have to think about the idea of eating menstrual blood as well. Menstruating women can be very powerful in sexual magick. It seems the menses open up access into the higher planes; or perhaps elemental spirits are attracted by the blood. In either case, menstrual blood in the resulting fluids of sex seems to add great efficacy to your work. Aleister Crowley likes to refer to this as the red elixir, or red gold.

If you have done your working with power and integrity, the resulting fluids will have a sweet and unique taste that is not at all repulsive. Somehow, an alchemical transformation takes place. This may be partly psychological, but it makes the sexual fluids into something other than residue. It truly is the elixir of life, the stone of the philosophers, the potable gold, the wine of the Sabbath of the adepts. In this age of STDs, particularly HIV, however, I suggest that you be aware of your partner's sexual health. And if you are seriously concerned about a potential partner's HIV status, you should probably not be having sex with them at all. Nor should you engage in sex magick with a partner who you know is HIV positive. If this is an issue for you, or if you really can't bear the thought of consuming even healthy fluids, you can simply apply them to your body, preserve them in a container, or use them on a talisman. There is an amazing power in this god-eating though. Ask any really devout Catholic.

Talismanic Magick

A talisman is an object that has been imbued with magical power. Talismanic magick is a very common practice among sex magicicians. The reason for this is simple. Since you create a living spiritual force, or incarnate a "magical child" with thaumaturgic sex magick, it is natural to want to give this child a "body" in the form of some physical object. At the end of the rite, the magically charged sexual fluids or some portion of them are placed on or in this object, thus vivifying it with magical force. This is an efficient and ancient procedure. You can also charge talismans autoerotically, however the energies are always more powerful when working with your lover.[53]

One of the convenient aspects of talismanic work is that, during the sex act, you need only concentrate upon the image of the talisman itself. You don't need to think about anything else, because your intention will be understood by your unconscious directly through the symbolic representation. If you have performed preliminary ritual invocations, so much the better! A mere thought about your talisman will bring all of your previous work to bear on the sexual energies you arouse.

There are many different ways to approach sex-magical talismans. Magicians use simple objects as talismans: a coin to manifest money, or sexual fluids on a picture to influence someone, or fluids on an object belonging to someone they want to influence. These are examples of "magical links," and these kinds of practices are often problematic, even if they work for you. However, ethics aside, this sort of simple procedure is extremely effective and you need not concern yourself with the more complicated methods outlined below unless you wish to. You may also magically charge rings, stones, charms, or other pieces of jewelry with the same procedure.

Most magicians like to make things slightly more complicated, however. Magical symbols connoting many layers of magical wisdom and knowledge of many ancient languages and writing scripts abound in most magicians' work. Symbols carved or carefully painted upon wood, metal, stone, papyrus, or parchment excite the imagination, and may lend themselves to greater efficacy for this very reason. If you feel as if your talisman is magical, well that's half the work done right there. Your subconscious mind will facilitate the work if excited by it. And funny symbols and mysterious ciphers stimulate the subconscious and the deeper strata of consciousness.

Though the medieval grimoirists, and even perhaps the Golden Dawn adepts, would probably like to tell you differently, there really isn't a correct or incorrect way to make a talismanic object. They are entirely personal creations—the result of an interaction between various layers of your consciousness to make an image that represents your desired outcome.

MONOGRAM SIGILS

One of the most efficient ways to make a talisman is to sigilize a sentence of desire—a method popularized by Chaos Magick.[54] First, create a sentence that expresses what you want. The statement must be a positive affirmation of what you desire. "My girlfriend will call me." Then remove all of the repeating letters from the sentence. These garbled letters of your sentence of desire can also be used as the basis of a mantra to keep you focused throughout your sex-magick rite. Using the phrase "My girlfriend will call me," the process looks like this:

MY GIRLFRIEND WILL CALL ME

MY GIRLF★★END W★★★ CA★★ ★★

MYGIRLFENDWCA

Combine the remaining letters into a single composite symbol that "looks magical" to you. This can be done in an infinite number of ways, but try to keep your sigil reasonably simple so you can call it clearly to mind when you charge it with your sex magick. The example above might look like this:

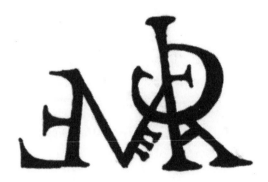

Figure 17. Sigilization of "My girlfriend will call."

Once you've developed a symbol that you find appealing, you can turn it into a talisman constructed of whatever material you like. You can carve it, paint it, sculpt it, or merely use the scrap of paper on which you first drew it. You are the best person to set your own magical requirements. You can add other magical symbols if you like, or color the talisman in an appropriate color related to the energy of your desire. For instance, the above might be colored green to connect with the energies of Venus.

You may also use complementary colors—often called "flashing colors" because, when you stare at them, they begin to reverse themselves, creating strange optical effects. These pairs of complementary colors are red and green, blue and orange, yellow and purple, and black and white. Make the background of your talisman one color, and make the symbol itself its flashing complement.

You may even use much simpler general concepts to create mono-gram sigils. You don't have to create a full sentence. For the above desire, I could simply use the word "call" and create a sigil for that. If I desired material opulence, I might create a sigil from the word "wealth." You can also forego language altogether and create an ideogram instead of a sentence. It's all really a matter for your own creativity.

MAGICAL SCRIPTS

Another way you can make talismans "magical" is to use an ancient script, either as the basis of a monogram, or simply by writing out your desire in a magical script. Figure 18 gives several popular magical scripts, and some monogram sigils based on the sentence above.

THE ROSE CROSS AND PLANETARY KAMEA

Another interesting way to develop a talisman, either based on a sen-tence of desire or any other representative word or appropriate spirit, is to trace a sigil upon the Golden Dawn Rose, or one of the Planetary Kamea. These symbols represent universal archetypal energies in a unique and powerful way, based on the Hebrew Qabala and its numerol-ogy. The Golden Dawn Rose is based on the ancient relationships between the Hebrew letters and astrology, as found in the *Sepher Yetzirah* (see figure 19).

The Planetary Kamea are numerical ciphers, in which the columns and rows equal the magical numbers of each of the planets. Figure 20, for instance, gives the Kamea of Venus. The numbers proceed numer-ically from one to the magical number squared, and all columns and rows add up to the same value, no matter which way you add them. Sigils traced on these magical cipher-symbols often look fairly odd, but they have the advantage of "magical significance."

The Golden Dawn Rose is a universal symbol that can be used for any purpose, while the Planetary Kamea obviously have individual pur-poses congruent with the planetary energies. In order to use these sym-bols, you must transliterate your letters into Hebrew, then inscribe the sigil. Figure 21 shows the resulting sigil, traced on the Golden Dawn Rose. This symbol could form the center of a talisman.

In order to trace this or any other symbol on a Planetary Kamea, you must convert the letters into numbers. Luckily, Hebrew letters have always also represented numbers, so this is easy enough to do. Using

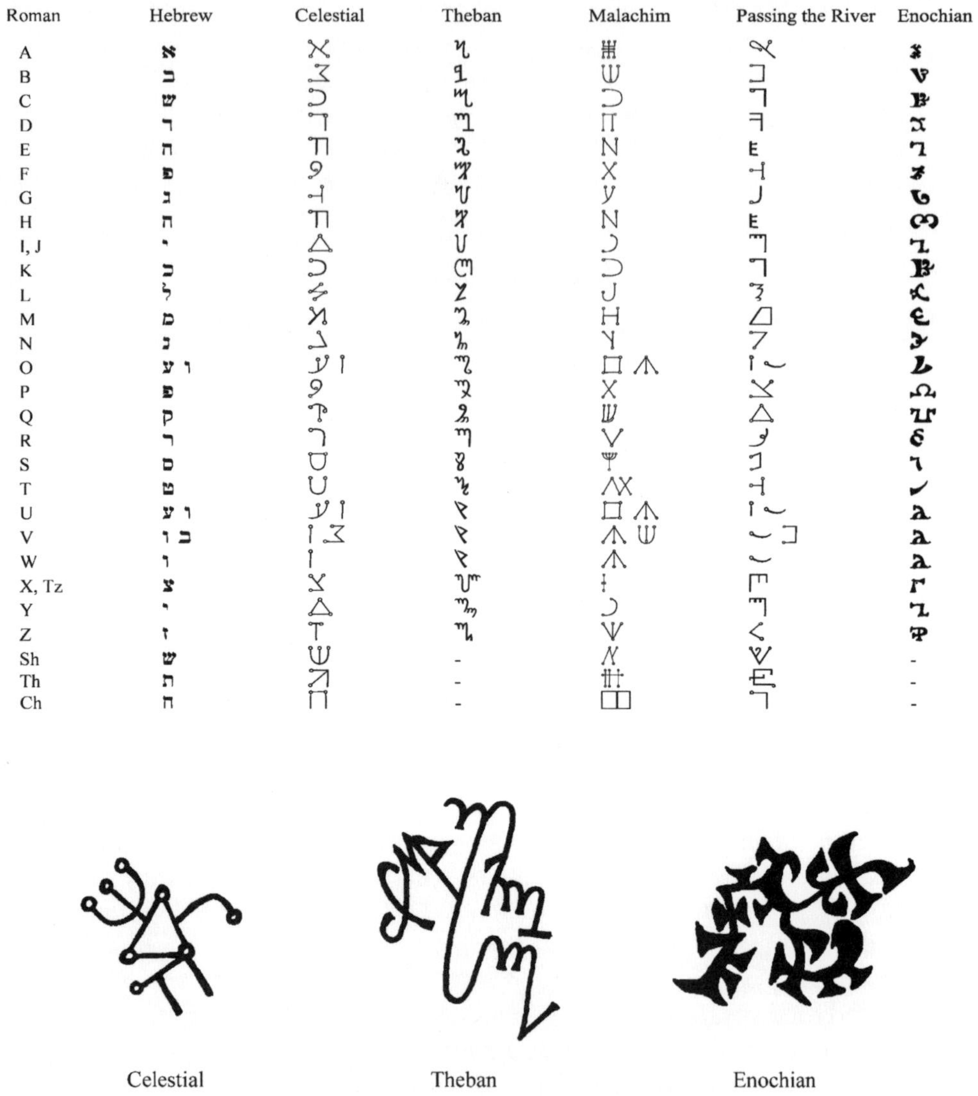

Roman	Hebrew	Celestial	Theban	Malachim	Passing the River	Enochian
A	א					
B	ב					
C	ג					
D	ד					
E	ה					
F	ו					
G	ז					
H	ח					
I, J	י					
K	כ					
L	ל					
M	מ					
N	נ					
O	ע					
P	פ					
Q	ק					
R	ר					
S	ס					
T	ט					
U	ע					
V	ו					
W						
X, Tz	צ					
Y	י					
Z	ז					
Sh	ש			-		-
Th	ת			-		-
Ch	ח			-		-

Celestial   Theban   Enochian

Figure 18. Magical scripts and sample sigilizations

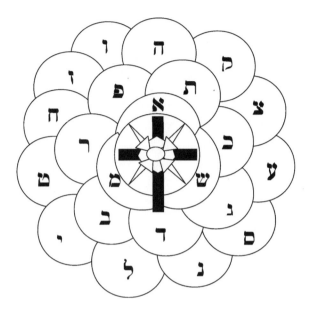

Figure 19. The Golden Dawn Rose

22	47	16	41	10	35	4
5	23	48	17	42	11	29
30	6	24	49	18	36	12
13	31	7	25	43	19	37
38	14	32	1	26	44	20
21	39	8	33	2	27	45
46	15	40	9	34	3	28

Figure 19. The Golden Dawn Rose

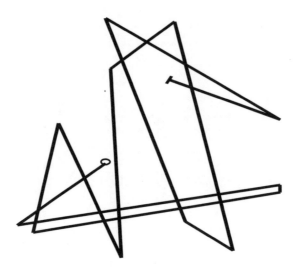

Figure 21. Sigil traced on the Golden Dawn Rose

the values shown in figure 22, the resulting numbers for our sentence of desire are:

M	Y	G	I	R	L	F	E	N	D	W	C	A
40	10	3	10	200	30	80	6	50	4	5	20	1

Because this desire falls under the influence of Venus, trace it on her Kamea. The resulting sigil is displayed in figure 23.

The observant will note that the numbers on the Kamea of Venus go no higher than forty-nine, while there are several higher figures in our phrase. Luckily, the ancient Hebrew magi already thought themselves out of this conundrum with another magical cipher system called *AIQ BKR*, or the Qabala of Nine Chambers. In this system, all of the letters sharing similar numbers are grouped (see figure 24). In the Kamea of Venus, the numbers can be reduced as follows: 4, 10, 3, 10, 20, 30, 8, 6, 5, 4, 5, 20, 1.

Sex and Visions–The Sleep of Siloam

The basic thaumaturgic sex-magick rite can also be adapted to accessing the higher planes and experiencing visions. Through it, you can achieve knowledge, inspiration, telepathic experiences, clairvoyance,

א	A – Aleph	1
ב	B – Beth	2
ג	G – Gimel	3
ד	D – Daleth	4
ה	H – Heh	5
ו	U, V, O – Vau	6
ז	Z – Zayin	7
ח	Ch – Cheth	8
ט	T – Teth	9
י	I, Y, J – Yod	10
כ	K, C – Kaph	20
ל	L – Lamed Libra	30
מ	M – Mem	40
נ	N – Nun	50
ס	S – Samekh	60
ע	O, A – Ayin	70
פ	P – Peh	80
צ	Tz – Tzaddi	90
ק	Q, K – Qoph	100
ר	R – Resh	200
ש	Sh – Shin	300
ת	Th – Tau	400
ך	K, C – Kaph final	500
ם	M – Mem final	600
ן	N – Nun final	700
ף	P – Peh final	800
ץ	Tz – Tzaddi final	900

Figure 22. Numerical values of the Hebrew letters

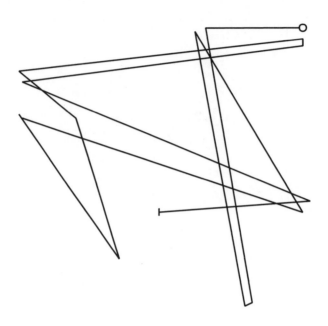

Figure 23. Sigil traced on the Kamea of Venus

ש ל ג	ר כ ב	ק י א
300, 30, 3	200, 20, 2	100, 10, 1
ם ס ו	ך נ ה	ת מ ר
600, 60, 6	500, 50, 5	400, 40, 4
ץ צ ט	ף פ ח	ן ע ז
900, 90, 9	800, 80, 8	700, 70, 7

Figure 24. AIQ BKR, the Qabala of Nine Chambers

and astral travel. To begin, you must clearly define the kind of experience you want to have in ceremonial invocations or whatever form of
preliminary preparations you prefer. For instance, if you want to obtain
a vision of the elemental plane of water, perform the appropriate pentagram rituals. If you wanted to obtain some hidden or arcane knowledge, create a preliminary statement of your intention and state it clearly
before the universe before you begin. Once you are in the ritual space
and having sex with your partner, there are two basic techniques for
achieving a visionary state:

> Prolong and extend your sex for an extremely long time, holding
> back orgasm through any of the techniques we've discussed.
> Continue holding out in this manner until you are in a
> profoundly altered state. This is the "borderland state" of the
> G∴B∴G∴. In this visionary state, you will obtain the
> information you desire.

> After an extended period of time, allow yourself to climax and, in
> the quiescent period after orgasm, melt into the same visionary
> state. You can also attempt Crowley's method of continuing the
> sexual stimulation until complete physical, emotional, and
> spiritual exhaustion launches you into a truly comatose visionary
> condition.

Your own experiences will suggest further modifications and you
will begin to create your own unique approaches with practice. These
same two principles will form the core of the practices we will discuss
in the next three chapters on invocation, evocation, and mysticism.

CHAPTER 7

Sexual Invocation, or Theurgy

But to love me is better than all things: if under the night-stars in the desert thou presently burnest mine incense before me, invoking me with a pure heart, and the Serpent flame therein, thou shalt come a little to lie in my bosom.

—*Liber AL vel Legis, I, 61*

One of the most powerful things that you can do with sexual magick is to invoke the higher-consciousness forms known collectively as "the gods." These ancient thought forms are archetypes that continue to inform our lives, though their temples have long since been razed to the ground. Their essence remains in our unconscious minds, and they continue to inspire art and poetry all over the world. The goddess of love, the god of war, the Sun and the Moon, the god of liars, thieves, and businessmen, the god of kings and leaders, the god of death and old age—these archetypes and many more form a part of our cultural heritage, and a part of our individual minds as well. By forming a conscious personal relationship with these archetypes, we gain their power and wisdom.

We have already explored invocation in the sexual practice of connecting with your Holy Guardian angel. But the gods are different from the Holy Guardian Angel, as they are completely universal in character. Your Holy Guardian Angel is universal in that it is your connection to the totality of consciousness, but it is also intimately personal because it is your own connection. Your Holy Guardian Angel is the axis of the wheel of your existence, while the ancient gods may be viewed more as the spokes of this wheel. They are those emanations from ultimate

Godhead that carry some unique, sublime, universal quality of existence. There are many reasons to invoke these gods. Among the most important is the need to understand the universe from an exalted perspective, to gain some missing piece of character or consciousness exemplified by a god, or to gain the power of a god to empower a magical operation.

Invocation from the perspective of sexual sorcery, however, entails more than just calling upon the gods themselves. It is an attempt to invoke any archetypal energy or quality into your life through sex. The following exercise gives a simple way to do just this. In many ways, this basic technique is the most powerful, because it goes directly to the root of the work, without any cultural or ideological baggage.

You can perform this exercise autoerotically or with a partner, though the instructions here describe working with a partner. You can easily adapt it, if you wish, for working alone. It is essentially the same as the thaumaturgic rite described earlier, but focuses entirely on you and/or your partner, and on the quality that you want to manifest in your life. It can be an excellent corrective for problems and limitations in your character. You can invoke courage, wisdom, beauty, trust, happiness, charisma, wit, or any other quality you would like to increase in your life.

Invoking Desired Qualities

1. Choose a specific quality you want to invoke into your being.
2. Get into a magick state of mind with your partner, using bathing, meditations, and/or rituals.
3. Ritually acknowledge what you are invoking. This can be done as formally or as informally as you like.
5. Stimulate each other sexually to full arousal, for the time being ignoring the purpose of the rite. It will remain in the background of your consciousness if you have properly formulated your intent.
6. Once you and your partner are completely aroused, begin having passionate and loving sex. Now focus your thoughts and your energies on the quality you are invoking, continuously visualizing that you are preparing to incarnate your force or desire. Your passionate connection with your partner is the path of manifestation for your desire. You can focus on the quality abstractly, or imagine it as a star of energy forming between you and your partner.

7. Let the sexual fires to be as ecstatic as possible. If you begin to lose your arousal, change your focus briefly to just the beauty and seductiveness of your partner to build up sexual energy. Then, as soon as you have recovered focus, redirect this energy toward your purpose.

8. Come to the edge of orgasm with your partner several times. Pull the energy inward and upward using one of the previous energy-movement techniques, concentrating on the quality all the time.

9. When you do yield to genital orgasm, try to climax at the same time as your partner and direct the purpose of the operation into that ecstasy together.

10. Gather the sexual fluids and consume them with your lover as a Eucharist. In eating the fluids, recognize that you are taking the energy of the rite into your bodies as a sacred communion with each other and the divine. The life of the operation is becoming a part of each of your lives. If the operation is specifically to benefit one operant only, he or she can eat all of the fluids alone.

11. Perform any closing rites, and record your experience in your journal.

Invocation of the Gods

In order to form a relationship with a god, you must understand as much as you can about the nature of that god. The Internet can be an excellent place to start your explorations. The god you choose may be of the opposite or the same sex, as long as it is a god toward whom you can feel sexually and spiritually drawn. Table 9 gives the names of some of the gods and goddesses who are commonly invoked in sex magick.

Table 9. Sexual God and Goddess Names

Sexual Goddesses

Aphrodite	Freya	Nuit
Astarte	Hera	Parvati
Babalon	Innanna	Shakti
Baphomet	Ishtar	Sophia
Ennoia	Isis	Venus

Sexual Gods

Baphomet	Eros	Mercury
Chaos	Frey	Shiva
Christos	Jupiter	Thor
Dionysus	Logos	Zeus
Dumuzi	Mars	

When choosing a god to invoke, find one that has qualities or characteristics you feel are lacking in yourself. Choose a god that connects in some way with work you are presently conducting on yourself, or one who has knowledge, power, or insight into something you desire to understand more fully. Either way, your intention should be to add something new to your life through interaction with this archetypal being.

Once you have chosen a god to invoke, consider yourself a devoted worshipper of this god, and dedicate yourself to living a life in harmony with its will. Think about the god often, setting up a shrine in your bedroom and/or in your dedicated temple space. The shrine should hold an image of your god that is both sublime and sexually stimulating. You may have to construct this image yourself. Figure 25 gives an example of what to aim for in this image.

Once you have become a devotee of your chosen god, you can begin performing rites as often as you like to connect more fully to this god sexually. You will probably have to do repeated work to get a profound result. You may choose to reach physical climax during these rites, or not. It is up to you. If you do choose to climax, give any resulting fluids to your god, either by placing them in a container in your shrine, or by anointing the image of your god directly.

Invoking the Gods Autoerotically

1. Enter a magick trance.
2. Perform whatever opening ritual elements you prefer, including purification, consecration, oaths, or ceremonial invocations.
3. Sit or lie down, and relax your body and mind fully.
4. When you are in a relaxed and concentrated state, begin to stimulate yourself sexually until you are fully aroused.

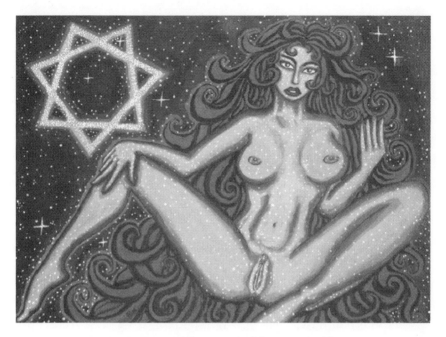

Figure 25. Invoking image of the Star Goddess

5. Masturbate ardently, invoking union with the god or goddess of your choice, visualizing it vividly before you. You do not need to visualize yourself having sex with your god. Just imagine yourself face to face with an erotic image of Godhead, then seek connection with it.

6. As you draw near to orgasm, progressively move the energy up into you, while focusing on the god form. Allow it to come closer and closer to you; feel it become more and more intimate and powerfully connected with you. Repeat this process as often as you like. Throughout, concentrate lovingly on your devotion to and love for this god. Give yourself to your god as completely as you can.

7. Continue stimulating yourself, moving the energy up to your belly, your chest, your throat, your head. Draw this out as long as you can.

8. Become totally enveloped in the light and love of your god. Feel yourself dissolving ecstatically into the light. You may yield to physical orgasm or not, depending on your personal feelings. If you do yield to orgasm, be certain that your mind is filled completely with your god as you climax. At first, it may be best not to climax. Instead, fill yourself and dissolve more and more with each near-climax, never yielding fully to physical release. This may cause you to dissolve completely into ecstasy.

9. Experience this state for as long as you like. Return to normal consciousness and perform closing rituals whenever you are ready.

10. If you have climaxed, give the consecrated sexual fluids to your god.

11. Record your results in your journal.

Repeat this process over time until union is complete. Once you have experienced a profound union with your chosen god, stop working with it, or you may become obsessed with it and lose focus on other work. You can start working with another god, or work on something else entirely. It may help to set a time limit—perhaps a month—for working with a particular god form, so that you don't risk feeling "stuck" in the relationship.

The next exercise is perhaps best performed with two partners who assume the form of a divine pair and make love as gods. This honors your partner and avoids using him or her as a surrogate for some divine fantasy lover.

You can also perform a sexual invocation with one partner acting as the god, and the other assuming the role of a mortal devotee. This sort of work is quite common historically, particularly with women acting as avatars for the goddess for male aspirants. Either method can result in profound and transformative experiences.

The singular devotee approach has certain advantages over working an invocation in unison with your partner. It is an invocation of one God form, with both partners gaining the power and wisdom of the same God. This will help to focus the energy. One partner gets to literally "be" the god, while the other gets to worship and unite with that god. When invoking together, you may wish to give an offering of food, wine, or incense to the god, and worship your partner as the god in a conventional sense before beginning any sex rite.

Invoking the Gods with Your Lover

1. Enter a magick trance with your partner, and perform whatever opening ritual elements you prefer, including purification, consecration, oaths, or ceremonial invocations.
2. Assume the god form(s) you have chosen, and arouse each other lovingly, worshipfully invoking the energy of your chosen god(s).
3. When you are both fully aroused, begin to make love.
4. Once you are blissfully intermingled, focus completely on experiencing the magical union. You may, as in other work, repeatedly bring yourself to near-climax, each time directing the sexual energy toward a more complete connection with the divine forces.
5. After prolonged lovemaking, you may climax or not, as you choose. Consider any sexual fluids produced divine, and treat them accordingly.
6. Record your results in your journal.

For an interesting alternative, try invoking deities of the opposite sex from you and your partner—the male invoking a goddess and the female invoking a god. Experience divine union in a counterbalanced sex rite. This, of course, may require a good deal of imagination and creativity. Sex toys might play a prominent role in such a rite!

A variation on sexual invocation that has a practical focus is the invocation of gods for specific magical purposes. The planetary gods are perfect for this sort of work, and some of the magical possibilities of such a rite are described in chapter 3. In the following exercise, one lover assumes the role of the operative god, while the other becomes a devotee or consort.

Invoking Planetary Gods

1. Enter a magick trance. After conducting any preliminary invocations and opening rituals, visualize the form of the appropriate planetary god in front of you. Give your visualization the characteristic pose and distinctive form of the god you have chosen. See this form glowing intensely, with an appropriately colored energy if you wish.
2. If you are the partner assuming the role of the god, move into the same position as the god in your visualization.

3. With your partner, imagine the form of the god moving into and encompassing you.

4. Expand your consciousness into the consciousness of the god, becoming the god as much as possible. If you are working with a divine pair, repeat this process with the other lover.

5. Arouse each other lovingly, worshipfully invoking the energy of your chosen god(s).

6. When you are both fully aroused, begin to make love.

7. Begin to focus your thoughts and energies on the purpose of the operation, continuously visualizing the incarnation of your force or desire.

8. Together, come to the edge of orgasm several times, pulling the energy inward and upward using one of the previous energy-movement techniques. You can make the number of times you do this correspond with the nature of the operation—with the planetary numbers, for instance. Draw this ecstasy out as long and as passionately as possible.

9. As you climax with your partner, visualize that it is the god who climaxes, and that the energies of the god are incarnated in the sexual fluids produced.

10. Gather the sexual fluids and place them on a talisman or on a "magical link" if you have one. Consume the rest with your partner as a Eucharist. As you both eat the fluids, recognize that you are taking the energy of the rite into your bodies as a sacred communion—with each other and with the divine. The operation becomes a part of each of you. If you are working to benefit only one partner, that person can eat all of the fluids alone.

11. Perform any closing rites. Be sure to reverse the invocation, imagining the energy of the god disconnecting from you. Thank the god for participating.

12. Record your experience in your journal.

The Tarot Archetypes

The tarot trumps make wonderful archetypes for invocation work, because they are so varied and their energies are so definitively part of a clear plan for personal evolution. I have found the tarot archetypes extremely useful, both in practical magick and in understanding my own inner universe. Each card contains multiple archetypal ideas, as well as correspondences to astrology, alchemy, Gnosticism, and the ancient mysteries, making them a rich source of both inspiration and power. Below I give a summary of these archetype and correspondences.

There are three ways to work with the tarot from a sexual perspective. You can approach it autoerotically, work with a partner, or conduct your work entirely in your body of light, keeping any sexual interaction on a purely imaginary or energetic level. This is the method I use most often, and it is this method that we will now discuss. As for the other two methods, you can easily adapt the techniques discussed earlier in this chapter to sexual workings with the tarot.

When you work with these archetypes through your imagination, you can still produce profound physiological effects, even though you don't involve your genitalia directly in the work. I have had numerous powerful "kundalini-awakening" experiences as a result of working with the tarot figures on a purely imaginary and energetic level.

THE WORLD (THE UNIVERSE)

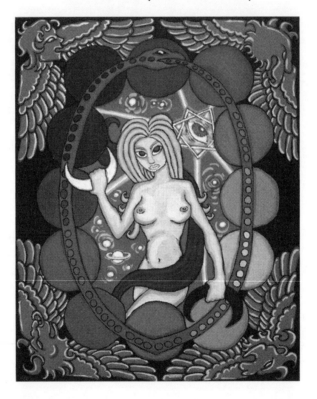

Key number: 21
Title: The Great One of the Night of Time
Inner experience: exploring the aethyr
Archetypal ideas: anima mundi, dancer, æthyr, astral light, four
    elements, material world, universe, maiden, initiatrix
Hebrew letter: Tau "Th"
Astrological correspondence: Earth, Saturn
Color: Indigo

THE LAST JUDGMENT

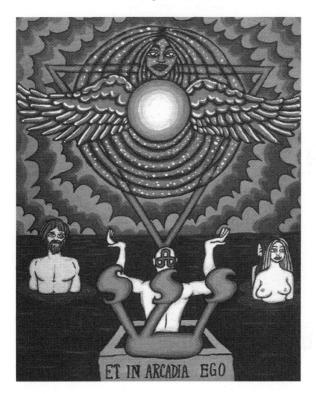

Key number: 20
Title: The Spirit of the Primal Fire
Inner experience: death and rebirth
Archetypal ideas: resurrection, baptism, eternal life, apocalypse,
     Hades, ecstasy, release
Hebrew letter: Shin "Sh"
Astrological correspondence: fire, spirit
Color: glowing orange, scarlet

THE SUN

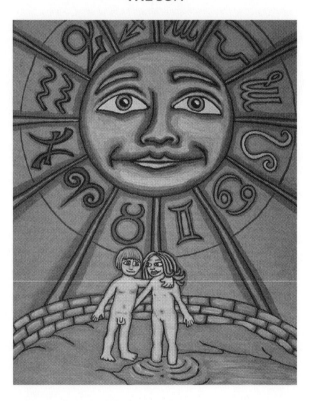

Key number: 19
Title: The Lord of the Fire of the World
Inner experience: invoking light of self
Archetypal ideas: self, ego, day, animus, extrovert, youth, child,
   aesthete, performer, left brain, solar powers, energy
Hebrew letter: Resh "R"
Astrological correspondence: Sun
Color: orange

THE MOON

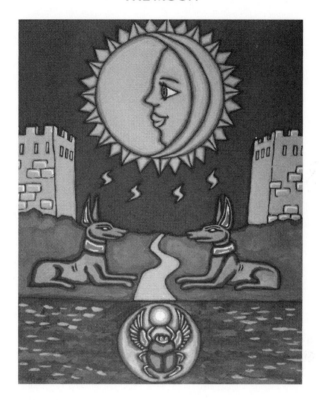

Key number: 18

Titles: The Ruler of Flux and Reflux, The Child of the Sons of the
Mighty

Inner experience: past lives, archetypes

Archetypal ideas: illusions, dreams, night, subconscious,
unconscious, fantasy, mystic, trance, right brain

Hebrew letter: Qoph "Q"

Astrological correspondence: Pisces

Color: crimson (ultra-violet)

THE STAR

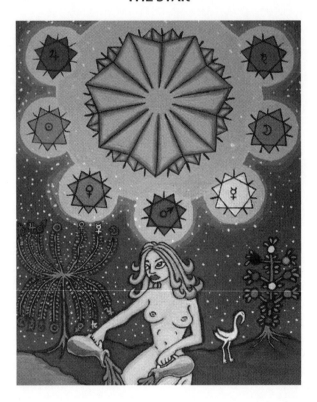

Key number: 17
Titles: The Daughter of the Firmament, The Dweller Between the
   Waters
Inner experience: expanding consciousness
Archetypal ideas: meditation, revelation, nature's beauty,
   imagination, scientist, freedom, unfolding of creation
Hebrew letter: Tzaddi "Tz"
Astrological correspondence: Aquarius
Color: violet

THE TOWER

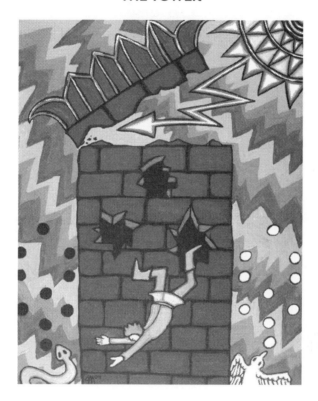

Key number: 16
Title: The Lord of the Hosts of the Mighty
Inner experience: silencing thought
Archetypal ideas: nature's power, Tower of Babel, dark night of
    soul, phallic energy, catastrophe, eye of Shiva
Hebrew letter: Peh "P"
Astrological correspondence: Mars
Color: scarlet

THE DEVIL

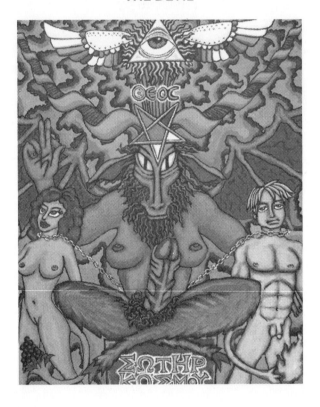

Key number: 15
Titles: The Lord of the Gates of Matter, The Child of the Forces of
    Time
Inner experience: talismanic work
Archetypal ideas: Pan, matter, material force, world father,
    Baphomet, demiurge, Satan, oppressor, redeemer
Hebrew letter: Ayin "O"
Astrological correspondence: Capricorn
Color: indigo

TEMPERANCE

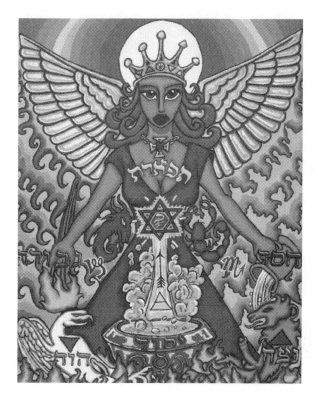

Key number: 14
Titles: The Daughter of the Reconcilers, The Bringer-Forth of Life
Inner experience: rising on the planes
Archetypal ideas: alchemy, teacher, guide, art, guardian angel, Great
    Work, transformer, philosopher
Hebrew letter: Samech "S"
Astrological correspondence: Sagittarius
Color: blue

DEATH

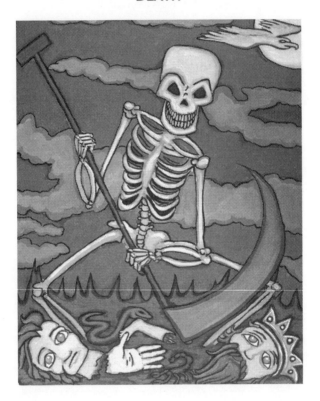

Key number: 13
Titles: The Child of the Great Transformers, The Lord of the Gate of
    Death
Inner experience: transcendence
Archetypal ideas: angel of death, transformation, snake, scorpion,
    eagle, reincarnation, reproduction, completion
Hebrew letter: Nun "N"
Astrological correspondence: Scorpio
Color: green-blue

THE HANGED MAN

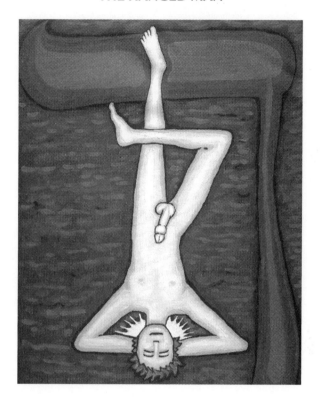

Key number: 12
Title: The Spirit of the Mighty Waters
Inner experience: power through sacrifice, radiating love
Archetypal ideas: sacrifice, illumination, crucifixion, masochist,
    victim, martyr, beneficence, dissolution
Hebrew letter: Mem "M"
Astrological correspondence: water
Color: deep blue

STRENGTH

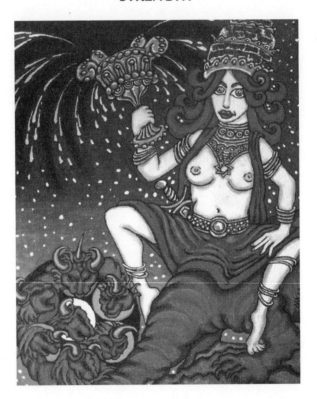

Key number: 11
Title: The Daughter of the Flaming Sword
Inner experience: learning to use power
Archetypal ideas: lover, power, vitality, lust, domination, strength of
    love, sorceress, fascination
Hebrew letter: Teth "T"
Astrological correspondence: Leo
Color: greenish yellow

THE WHEEL OF FORTUNE

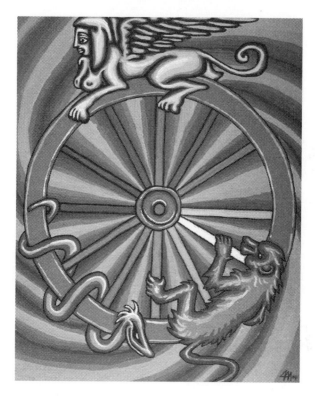

Key number: 10
Title: The Lord of the Forces fo Life
Inner experience: undoing past experience
Archetypal ideas: luck, karma, fate, gambler, cycles, wealth and
    luck, chance, expansion, success
Hebrew letter: Kaph "K"
Astrological correspondence: Jupiter
Color: violet

THE HERMIT

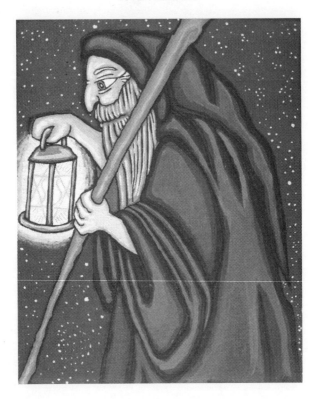

Key number: 9
Titles: The Prophet of the Eternal, The Magus of the Voice of Power
Inner experience: absorbing power
Archetypal ideas: loner, sage, path of initiation, pilgrim, inner
    knowledge, secret seed, secret light
Hebrew letter: Yod "I, J, Y"
Astrological correspondence: Virgo
Color: yellowish green

JUSTICE

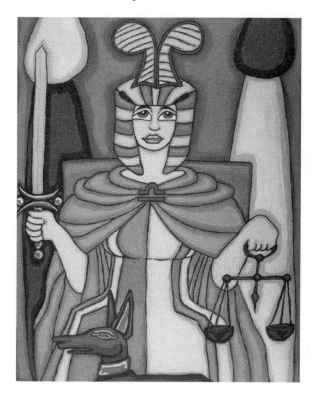

Key number: 8
Titles: The Daughter of the Lords of Truth, The Ruler of the
    Balance
Inner experience: balancing forces
Archetypal ideas: balance, karma's action, balance of opposites,
    judge, adjustment, equilibrium, mediator, truth
Hebrew letter: Lamed "L"
Astrological correspondence: Libra
Color: emerald green

THE CHARIOT

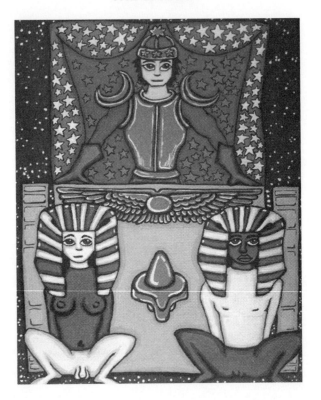

Key number: 7
Titles: The Child of the Powers of the Waters, The Lord of the
     Triumph of Light
Inner experience: giving all for wisdom
Archetypal ideas: grail bearer, receptivity, reconciliation, transport,
     the ark, containment
Hebrew letter: Cheth "Ch"
Astrological correspondence: Cancer
Color: amber

THE LOVERS

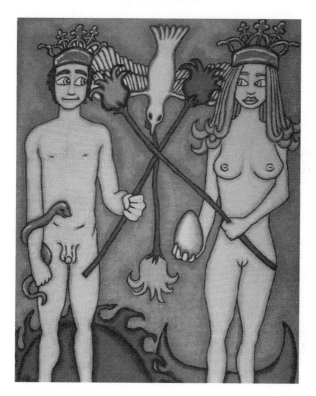

Key number: 6

Titles: The Children of the Voice, The Oracle of the Mighty Gods

Inner experience: The Chymical Wedding

Archetypal ideas: twins, lovers, attraction of opposites, polarity, two halves of the brain

Hebrew letter: Zayin "Z"

Astrological correspondence: Gemini

Color: orange

THE HIEROPHANT

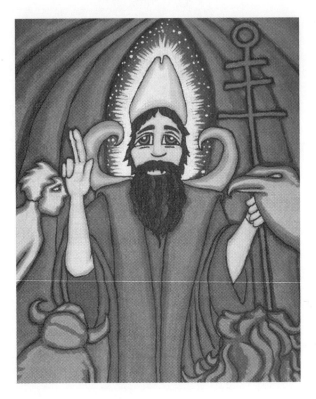

Key number: 5
Title: The Magus of the Eternal
Inner experience: power to initiate
Archetypal ideas: master, teacher, high priest, spiritual rules or laws,
    interpreter of the mysteries
Hebrew letter: Vau "V, U"
Astrological correspondence: Taurus
Color: red–orange

THE EMPEROR

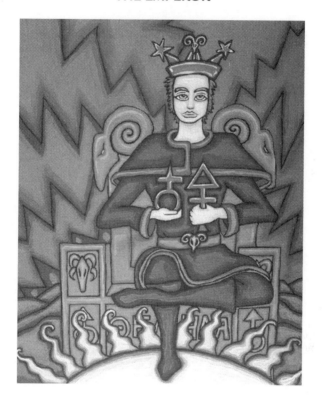

Key number: 4
Titles: The Son of the Morning, Chief Among the Mighty
Inner experience: cosmic strength
Archetypal ideas: all-father, conqueror, father, creator gods,
    husband, alchemical sulfur, warrior
Hebrew letter: Heh "H"
Astrological correspondence: Aries
Color: scarlet

THE EMPRESS

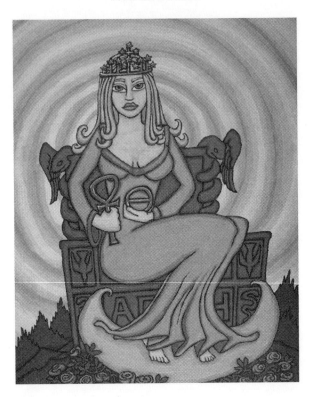

Key number: 3
Title: The Daughter of the Mighty Ones
Inner experience: cosmic love
Archetypal ideas: Mother Nature, the beauty of nature, mother, manifester, love, wife, Demeter, queen, goddess, alchemical salt
Hebrew letter: Daleth "D"
Astrological correspondence: Venus
Color: emerald green

THE HIGH PRIESTESS

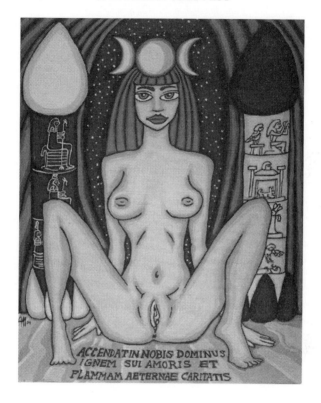

Key number: 2
Title: The Priestess of the Silver Star
Inner experience: divine presence
Archetypal ideas: priestess, wise woman, yoni, gnosis, Isis, the
    hidden sanctuary, beauty
Hebrew letter: Gimel "G"
Astrological correspondence: Moon
Color: blue

THE MAGICIAN

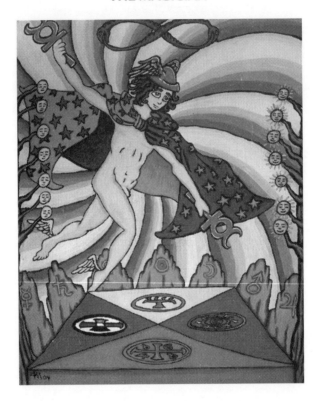

Key number: 1
Title: The Magus of Power
Inner experience: cosmic knowledge
Archetypal ideas: Prometheus, trickster, wizard, inventor, artist, creative will, magick power, Hermes
Hebrew letter: Beth "B"
Astrological correspondence: Mercury
Color: yellow

THE FOOL

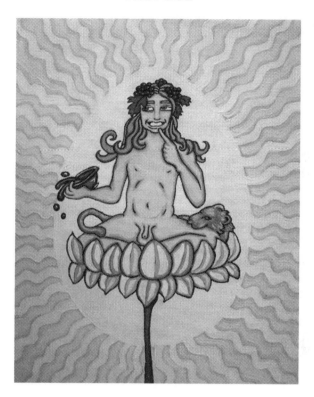

Key number: 0
Title: The Spirit of αιΘηρ
Inner experience: cosmic ecstasy
Archetypal ideas: divine folly, jester, joker, Babe in the Egg, the
    Green Man, spirit, chaos, mad genius, Dionysus
Hebrew letter: Aleph "A"
Astrological correspondence: air
Color: bright pale yellow

These figures can be split conveniently into male, female, and gender-neutral energies fairly easily, though some may be ambiguous. Table 10 gives my interpretation of this distribution.

Note that nearly all of the male cards are definite characters that can easily be placed in a context. Of the female cards, only two have clear human personas; the rest represent lofty principles or celestial bodies that are more ideals than personalities. This is a really good example of how, for centuries, women have been put up on a mystical and philosophical pedestal of virtue, while in reality they have been ill-defined and consigned to menial roles. Still, we can discover the truth within the archetypes, because the images themselves and the cosmic energies at play behind them tell a story that can be quite different from the names on the card.

Table 10. Gender Distribution of Tarot Archetypes

Female Tarot Cards	High Priestess
	Empress
	Lust/Strength
	Adjustment/Justice (could also be neuter)
	Art/Temperance (could also be neuter)
	The Star
	The Moon
	The Universe
Male Tarot Cards	The Fool
	The Magician
	The Emperor
	The Hierophant
	The Hanged Man
	Death
	The Devil
	The Sun
Gender-neutral Tarot Cards	The Lovers
	Fortune (can also be male)
	The Chariot
	The Tower (can also be male)
	Aeon/Last Judgment

Active Imagination and the Tarot Archetypes

Because the tarot archetypes are accessible, they provide an excellent starting place for beginners who want to work with gods or other beings. You will want to work with all of the tarot archetypes over time, however, to fully understand the completeness of this system. You don't have to have astral sex with every single archetype. Some may not be interested in sexual interaction with you; others may not interest you sexually. One great advantage of tarot work, moreover, is that it provides a relatively safe atmosphere for working sexually with same-sex archetypes, and this may be important to some people.

Some tarot cards do not have a central figure. When working with these, allow a representative figure to appear at your call—one that is the living essence of the card. Generally, you should not force your experiences of the archetypes to conform to the images in the cards. By calling upon the energies of each card and accepting whatever form comes to you, you gain a deeper understanding of yourself and your inner world. For instance, when I first started using this technique, the Sun appeared to me as a very small and dull child, showing me that my self-esteem at the time was very low. By working with the figure, asking it what it wanted, and learning how to interact with it more positively, I discovered how to improve my own sense of self-worth.

I have had truly powerful experiences with nearly all of these imaginal figures, and this work has really influenced my life, helping me to evolve very rapidly and positively. Experience these archetypes for yourself, and experience sexual union with them wherever it is appropriate.

Invoking Sexual Archetypes

1. Enter a magick trance. You may also purify, consecrate, and cast a circle, or perform the Lesser Ritual of the Pentagram to get into the magical space.
2. Perform an appropriate pentagram or hexagram ritual to invoke the corresponding energy of the card, if you have an understanding of the astrological correspondences (see Table 7). This is not required, however.
3. Transfer your awareness to your body of light and travel upward, calling upon the energy of the card. Imagine yourself traveling through a tunnel of energy in the corresponding color of the card (see Table 3.)

4. At the end of the tunnel, visualize the card itself as a gateway into another realm. Travel through the card, entering the environment of this image.

5. As the scene unfolds before you, integrate yourself into it, whatever it may be. It may or may not resemble the traditional landscape of the card. Whatever appears is appropriate for you. Call upon the central figure of the card to appear.

6. When the figure appears to answer your call, it may or may not be familiar. It may also change appearance or shape over the course of your interaction. All of this is fine. The way in which it appears to you will communicate information about the archetype. Is it healthy? Sad? Energetic?

7. Ask the figure to communicate with you, and wait until you feel it has responded affirmatively. Ask the figure to tell you how you can get along with it most beneficially. Ask it how it feels about you, and your life, and your current sex partner. Ask if it has any advice for you. Ask if it will help you accomplish your goals, and work with you in the transformation of your life.

8. The communication may seem to come from a voice outside your consciousness, or it may seem to be in your own head, in your own voice. Consider any thoughts that come up to be communication from this figure. However strange the communication appears to be, thank the figure for relating to you.

9. If it seems appropriate, merge with the figure sexually, uniting your energy with its energy.

10. Thank the figure, and return back to your body.

11. Perform a banishing Lesser Ritual of the Pentagram, or simply return to normal consciousness.

12. Record your experience in your journal, and seriously consider any information that the archetypal figure related to you.

This simple technique can have profound results, particularly if the sexual interaction is powerful and vivid. Once you have sexually experienced tarot archetypes in this way, you can attempt to invoke them autoerotically or with your lover to ground the experience in physical expression. You can also direct archetypal energies magically, evoking their power using the method we will discuss in the next chapter.

CHAPTER 8

Sexual Evocation, or Goetia

Fear not at all; fear neither men nor Fates, nor gods, nor anything. Money fear not, nor laughter of the folk folly, nor any other power in heaven or upon the earth or under the earth.

—*Liber AL vel Legis, III, 17*

In chapter 7, we discussed invoking the higher qualities of gods and divine archetypes. In this chapter, we will explore using the sex act to evoke the lower elements of your cosmic being. In medieval times, the calling of spirits and the creation of artificial elementals or servitors was considered a dark art related to the conjuring of demons. Sexual liaisons with these creatures were considered congress with succubi and incubi. Our modern worldview allows us to see these creatures of darkness more as elements of consciousness—natural forces—rather than as servants of some chthonic arch-fiend dwelling in a fiery abyss.

These energies are really nothing more or less than a part of the function of the universe, both personally and generally. They are parts of your individual psyche, and of the general collective unconscious of humanity, and of the universe as a whole. They are hunger, desire, greed, anger, lust, murder, fear, ferocity, and all of the "unacceptable" aspects of nature that civilization has sought to eliminate from the human animal. But whether bestial or rudimentary, they are as much a part of you as the sublime archetypes of the gods. Rather than suppress these lower parts of your nature, you must redirect them toward your true aims in life. The tarot archetypes we just explored really partake of both qualities. We will focus here on directing the chaotic energies of the unconscious forces around you toward your True Will.

In many ways, sexual evocation resembles talismanic magick, both in theory and practice. In both, you direct a force to accomplish your desires. The only real difference is that, in one, you communicate with and treat your evoked beings as intelligences, while in the other, they operate as blind forces that you direct in a singular way. There are advantages and disadvantages to both, because, while the more sentient thought forms can be flexible, they can also take on a life of their own. Sometimes they may disobey you.

While, in a certain sense, these beings are just imaginary, they are a part of your inner world, and do have their own desires and wills. They are also, to a certain extent, perfectly real, even when they seem imaginary, and they do seem capable of effecting real change on consensus reality. You will continually be surprised.

Evocation of Spirits

There are several ways to approach evocation in sexual magick, just as with all of the other forms of sexual work we've discussed. You can work autoerotically, with a partner, or entirely within your body of light, just as with the archetypes. When working with negative spirits, however, it is usually a good idea to keep them at a distance from your spiritual body, so that they do not try to obsess you and usurp your dominance in the situation. This is why most medieval grimoires suggest evoking spirits into magical triangles outside the magical circle, or into magick mirrors or crystals.

The key is to remain in control when dealing with any entity, whether artificial or one whose name you've found in a book. Be on guard against trickiness, power plays, and uninvited appearances—in other words, always stay in charge of all your workings. If you evoke a spirit and it starts to misbehave, immediately banish it using ritual and your own mental fortitude. Do not let any situation get out of control.

So why would you want to conjure something that could become dangerous and out of control? Because these spirits are already a part of you, operating in the background of consciousness and life. By bringing them into your awareness, you can control and guide your relations with them and direct the contents of your own mind more consistently. By learning to control the demons of magick, you learn to control your own inner demons. Of course, you can also create all sorts of problems for yourself, but your wisdom and your own Holy Guardian

Angel will keep you out of trouble as long as you first concentrate on developing these relationships before involving yourself with any lower critters.

Most of your work with evocation should probably be in the form of creating your own artificial elementals and servitors, because these really tend to be the most practically useful, both in magical operations and in your own personal evolution. You are, after all, not really creating anything. Any artificial spiritual entity you evoke sexually already exists before you begin the working. You merely give shape and direction to energy and consciousness that is already flowing through your unconscious life and form a relationship with it.

Many people, on the other hand, enjoy working with spirits that have already been categorized, named, and classified. The most famous of these are the seventy-two demons of the *Lesser Key of Solomon the King*. You can also work with the nearly limitless spirits of the Enochian watchtowers, the spirits from *The Sacred Magic of Abramelin the Mage,* the planetary intelligences and spirits (see figure 26), or even the genii and *kakodemons* of the tarot, found in Crowley's *Holy Books of Thelema*. I have found beings from all of these hierarchies interesting, and they certainly have the advantage of already having defined functions.

There are two basic methods for evoking these beings. You can summon them, engaging in some sort of conversation using a magick mirror, or some other clairvoyance device or astral journey. Or you can use their seals in an almost talismanic way to direct them through thaumaturgic sex magick. This second method is much simpler and more straightforward, and you can use the techniques we've already discussed to do it.

Many people, on the other hand, prefer to hold long drawn-out conversations with these rather simple creatures of the unconscious. I don't really know why, since they rarely have anything particularly interesting to communicate, and often simply mirror the whims of the practitioners. It is a very popular sport among some magicians, however. Of course, there is really just as much to learn from these archetypes as any others. It is just a bit harder to get useful information from negative energy, although it is often easier to work with in other ways.

Evoking negative or lower spirits tends to be far easier than invoking gods or angels. They seem to respond fairly quickly to your call, often becoming immediately present the first time their names are mentioned. This is especially true when you involve blood or sex fluids in your work. These energies may not always manifest in an obvious

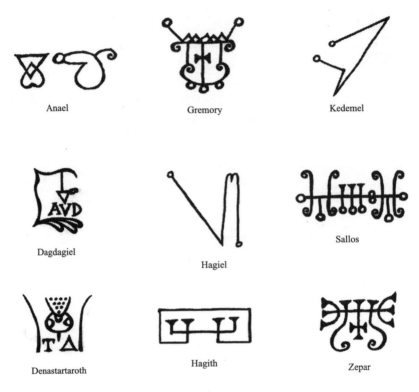

Anael

Gremory

Kedemel

Dagdagiel

Hagiel

Sallos

Denastartaroth

Hagith

Zepar

Figure 26. Examples of Venusian spirits

way, but they are invariably present before you even begin. They exist,
just like the other archetypal entities, within your own mind. At least
that's one way of looking at it. I have had a number of experiences in
which naughty spirits have sought to take control of a working, escaping from the triangle and refusing to leave when banished. These energies are certainly more than just fantasy.

When you work with these energies, stay in control, and maintain
a strict magical hygiene in your work. You may want to conduct this sort
of work with more ceremony than usual for this very reason. You will
also need some sort of magick mirror into which you can project these
entities. You can construct one by spray-painting a piece of glass black
to make it reflective, but dark. Visualize and communicate with the
entity through this mirror, or place it into a magick triangle like the
one shown in figure 27 outside your ceremonial circle.

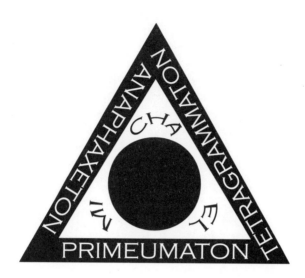

Figure 27. Triangle of Goetic evocation

You can evoke these spirits autoerotically or with a partner. You will discover advantages and disadvantages to both. If you work with a partner, choose one of you to enter directly into the communication, while the other acts as a guide and perhaps records the conversation—although this may be rather unsexy. This work is probably most easily conducted alone, though the energies will be stronger with a lover.

Evoking Spirits

1. Choose a spirit and draw its sigil or seal on a piece of paper, parchment, or metal, in appropriate color(s). You can draw this symbol on the magick mirror as well, and place it around your neck or the neck of your partner to help keep you focused on your intention.
2. If possible, work within a magical circle, and place your magick mirror in a conveniently visible spot outside the circle, within a triangle. If you work with a partner place the mirror so that you can see it clearly while astride your lover. Place the seal of the spirit within the magick triangle so that you can see both the mirror and the seal, and easily look back and forth between them.

3. Enter a magick trance, and perform whatever opening ritual elements you prefer, including purification, consecration, oaths, or ceremonial invocations.

4. For the moment, forget about the working and simply arouse yourself or each other lovingly for as long as you like, and then begin to masturbate or make love. The "seer"—the participant who is going to communicate directly with the spirit—should be on top, so that the mirror is easily visible. You can also use rear entry so that both participants can look at the mirror. But it is only necessary, and probably preferable, for one party to be the "seer."

5. Stimulate yourself to the edge of climax, pulling back at the point of no return, and draw in the ecstasy, directing it toward the seal and the magick mirror.

6. As you do, start your conjuration. You can use a traditional conjuration related to the spirit you are calling, or just something simple, like: "O mighty and powerful spirit _____, I conjure you very potently, appear in visible form before us in the magical triangle outside this Circle of Art."

7. You may need to repeat this process a few times, or you may feel contact immediately.

8. Once you feel that you have the attention of your spirit (this is an unmistakable sense of "contact"), begin your communications. Tell the spirit what you want it to do for you, or obtain whatever information you want.

9. Once you are sure that the spirit understands your intention, dismiss it, thanking it for participating and asking it to return to communicate more in the future if need be. Be sure that you see the figure dissolving away, or you can direct it into the seal in front of the mirror.

10. Finish the sex act, allowing yourself to climax, and directing the energy of the climax toward the spirit and the intention you have for it.

11. Gather up the sexual fluids and give them to the spirit by placing them on the seal. Wrap the seal in a black cloth.

12. Banish the energies of the spirit and make sure that you feel things have really cleared before ending your work. Perform any other closing rituals you desire.

13. Record your results in your journal.

You can also perform this working without ever climaxing, as an act of Dianism. Or you can climax before beginning your conversation, entering into a Sleep of Siloam at the end of your sexual intercourse to commune with the spirit. You will discover the method that is best for you through your own experimentation.

Artificial Elementals or Servitors

Artificial elementals or servitors are evoked beings that you create yourself. The great advantage of these talismanic beings is that they are distinctly your own creations and carry no cultural baggage. In my experience, however, their practical efficacy in accomplishing miraculous ends is comparable to that of any other evoked beings.

You can determine the exact function of these created beings and the type of energy you want them to contain. You can also determine their lifespan, so you can minutely control their existence and disintegration. Of course, each will have its own personality that emerges during your work, and this personality will not be chosen by you. These entities are part of your consciousness already; the evocation process merely brings them to the surface. When you disintegrate them, their component parts resume their previous place in your unconscious.

Some people like to create many short-term servitors to accomplish specific individual tasks. I prefer to create a limited number of long-term artificial elementals to serve as "familiar spirits" that I can direct toward whatever little tasks I like at any time. The following technique can easily be used for either purpose.

Crowley suggests four long-term familiars and that is the number of spirits that I have at my own disposal. The nice thing about this number is that it corresponds with the elements, so that I have a familiar for each elemental area: salamanders for fire, undines for water, sylphs for air, and gnomes for earth. I prefer this simple compartmentalized approach, because it makes things clear and leaves little room for confusion or fuzziness. You can also assign your familiars to the four times of the day: sunrise to noon, noon to sunset, sunset to midnight, and midnight to sunrise. This is what Abramelin suggests.

You can also use the names and functions of Enochian, planetary, or Qabalistic spirits or angels when creating familiars, servitors, or elementals. There is no wrong way to approach this. Just decide, before you begin to create it, its name, what its purpose will be, and how long it will remain alive and functional. If you create a servitor for a single specific purpose, you definitely want it to disintegrate immediately upon completing its task. Leaving a stray elemental floating about in your personal magical universe can cause any number of problems down the road. This is how obsessions begin.

When creating an artificial being sexually, choose an erotically stimulating image to embody your elemental. You may not necessarily have an astral affair with your elemental, but there's certainly no harm in making it attractive! The images of the Court cards of the tarot—particularly Crowley's Thoth Tarot— make excellent images to embody your elementals. Don't fall in love with your familiars, however. You bestow favor on them by giving them life, direction, and attention. Give your love to your gods or goddesses; give directions to your elementals and familiars.

Creating elemental servitors with a partner has an automatic advantage. Something subtle about the dynamics of partnership seems to lend power to beings created in this way. You create a magical child, and this makes your beings stronger by giving them the magical qualities of both "parents." Of course, when you create personal familiars you should probably work alone. It is quite simple to work either way.

Creating Artificial Elementals

1. Decide your elemental's purpose, its name, the amount of time it has to accomplish its mission, and the date on which it will terminate. (If it is a long-term or permanent familiar, obtain an appropriate material base—an image, picture, or sculpture—that can be its purified and consecrated home.

2. Enter a magick trance, and perform whatever opening ritual elements you prefer, including purification, consecration, oaths, or ceremonial invocations. If you use invocations, make sure that they invoke forces congruent with your elemental, either through ritual or some other means like simple visualization.

3. For the moment, forget about the working and simply arouse yourself or each other lovingly for as long as you like, and then begin to masturbate or make love.

4. Focus on the energy of your elemental all around you and draw it into you as you experience sexual pleasure—either your own masturbatory pleasure, or your passionate connection with your partner. This is the path of manifestation for this energy.

Concentrate on the energy and the task you are assigning the elemental.

5. Imagine the form of the elemental beginning to coalesce before you.

6. Come to the edge of orgasm several times, pulling the energy in and directing it into the elemental. The number of times you do this can correspond to the nature of the elemental, if this is appropriate. Let the ecstasy be as powerful as possible.

7. Yield to genital orgasm, directing the power of the orgasm into your elemental and its purpose.

8. Gather the fluids and either eat them or place them on the material base.

9. Perform any closing rites, and record your experience in your journal.

If you create long-term servitors or familiars, "feed" them occasionally with another sex rite and provide them with a physical home. Statues, figurines, and paintings all make excellent homes for elemental servitors. Just put the object in your vicinity when creating the elemental, and place your sexual fluids on it at the end of the rite.

Be on guard against the trickiness of your servitors. They may very quickly try to gain more power in your relationship, or refuse to do what they're asked. Be a firm but kind master. You are in command.

Artificial Succubae and Incubi

You can create an artificial elemental that will actually be a sort of dream lover. I have seen a number of variations on this technique over the years, but I found my own experiments in this direction to be rather creepy and I abandoned them. You may find the practice useful, nonetheless. These sorts of elementals are probably most useful when you don't have a physical human lover. They can help you focus your otherwise undirected sexual energy.

The danger in this practice is one of obsession. Both the practitioner and the entity can become obsessive. In fact, it is obsession itself that forms the basis of this work. Properly directed, this kind of entity can be magically potent, but I did not personally enjoy the interaction. You can create these entities using the previous technique, and then work with them using the next exercise. These are actually the steps I followed when I conducted my work in this area.

Creating Artificial Succubae and Incubi

1. Choose a sexually stimulating image to act as the focal point of your magical creation. This can be any stimulating image from your mind, or from an external source like a magazine, or from some combination of the two. You can name this entity, or just let it be a shadowy dream lover.
2. Each night as you fall asleep, focus on the entity. As you masturbate, crave the creature's presence, thinking of it with as much focused attention as you can.
3. Do not climax. Instead, let yourself fall asleep still thinking of your dream lover. Use any of the energy-moving techniques you like, but continually focus on attracting and devoting your energy toward this dream entity. Repeat this over many nights.
4. Eventually, in the half-sleep state, your magical entity will become a real presence, and you will feel its touch, hear its voice, and know its reality.
5. You can have sexual intercourse with this entity, and direct your will through this sex. This will be a half-physical, half-astral experience, and you will know it distinctly when it occurs.
6. Record your results in your journal.

This type of encounter may not happen every time you attempt it, but the more you devote yourself to the practice, the more often it will occur. Ultimately, you will be able to conduct any sort of magical work with this entity, from manifesting your desires to divining the future.

These entities can work quite a bit of practical magick for you, but they may become more and more of a nuisance as well. You may find yourself getting touched by them when you have not called them, and dreaming of them quite frequently. As long as you stay in control of the situation, however, it is probably not dangerous. Just use caution if you think you are becoming really obsessed.

CHAPTER 9

Sexual Mysticism

I give unimaginable joys on earth: certainty, not faith, while in
life, upon death; peace unutterable, rest, ecstasy; nor do I
demand aught in sacrifice.

—*Liber AL vel Legis, I, 58*

In many ways, sexual mysticism resembles "really good sex." The difference is that, while really good sex can be personally enlightening
and ecstatic, mystical sex merges your consciousness entirely into your
partner, and ultimately into universal consciousness, transcending the
personal altogether. Crowley describes it like this: "When the All is
absorbed within the I, it is as if the I were absorbed within the All; for
if two Things become wholly and indissolubly One Thing, there is no
more Reason for Names, since Names are given to mark off one Thing
from another."[55] We can transcend individual consciousness through
sex, overcoming our limitations and becoming one with our partner and
the universe in the act of sexual congress. This is the pathway of spiritual awakening and pure illumination, the path of the sexual mystic.

There is a common misconception that, somehow, the mystics of
our world permanently transcend the ordinary, shrugging off the bonds
of mortality and dwelling forever apart from the dross of humanity. On
the contrary, were it not for their great humanity, the mystics' accomplishments would be meaningless. It is their humanity that gives strength
to their conviction and their message. Were it not for Christ's humanity, his suffering on the cross would be meaningless. Were it not for the
humanity of the Buddha, his realizations under the Bodhi Tree would
be empty. How much more human, then, are the sexual mystics
who seek liberation through the very means denied by most mystical

methods. They descend into the midst of temptation and deny no urge, lust, or passion. Instead, they indulge all their senses and transcend through experience, rather than renunciation.

Mystics and saints are traditionally seen as putting aside normal life, foregoing sexuality and sense pleasures altogether. They are portrayed as people whose natures have shifted away from the mundane, who give up family life, money, and procreation and focus entirely on the spiritual side of life. This is a fairly modern convention, however. Old Testament mystics frequently had both wives and children. The hero of the *Bhagavad Gita* is a warrior on the eve of battle. The texts of Taoism refer to government and family affairs as much as direct spiritual instruction. Clearly, it is possible to conduct your spiritual life within the context of ordinary day-to-day existence.

Mystics do experience something outside of regular life, however—something transcendent, something formless. Both sexual mystics and those who withdraw from life share a unique experience of extraordinary knowledge. Both find something that leaves them forever altered, changed—though not necessarily forever beyond the mundane world.

We all experience small glimpses of the transcendent—in quiet times, dreams, drug experiences, and, yes, during sex. Nearly everyone has had some little taste of this divinely serene place. The only real difference between the mystic and the ordinary person is that the mystic considers this transcendent place to be the center of being, while the majority of humanity focuses on the individual ego. The mystic still possesses an ego, but sees it only as a function of consciousness rather than the whole of existence.

Transcendence and Liberation

Sexual mysticism is the same as any other mystical practice. Its intention is to slip behind the veil of ordinary existence to experience the transcendent face to face—or perhaps beyond faces. Sexual mystics obtain an experience of the eternal in which they realize that we are all at one with an omnipresent, omnipotent, omniscient, and timeless consciousness that has no beginning and no end. These experiences have nothing to do with morality, ethics, or life choices, so it is difficult to define the characteristics of a mystic. Indeed, these experiences entail a liberation from all qualifications and qualities.

This liberation comes, however, from a single phenomenon—the union of opposites and their transcendence. It comes, literally, as we move between these opposites at the intersection of their union. This is why sexuality is such a powerful path to transcendence. Sex abounds with opposites, consists of union, and presents a multitude of gateways between these opposing forces.

You find gateways to higher consciousness in "in-between" states: between thoughts and feelings, between sexual excitement and orgasm, between orgasm and quiescence, between breaths, between waking and sleeping, between thought and silence, between pain and pleasure, between effort and surrender. These are all states in which your true self, "the knower," your cosmic self, your ultimate consciousness, peeks through. In these moments, you realize your identity with infinity. And all of these states are easily available to you in every sexual experience.

Each of these moments is a gateway in which the totality of yourself is present. Jumping through the gateway brings you liberation. The way through the gateway is love, and this is something you must explore on your own. When you come to these gateways, you must find your own way through. There is no technique to give you a genuine, complete, and liberating mystical experience. It is something that comes of itself, when the time is right. All you can do is prepare the way. Any of the techniques in this book may lead to liberation and mystical transcendence if you make yourself available. By opening to love and real union with your lover, you make the gateway wider and the path clearer.

Let your love-making be unhurried. If you lose your drive because you are moving too slowly, stop for a little while. I know of a couple that felt bored while attempting to experience mystical sex. If this happens, you are missing the key ingredient: love. Let your connection be about your love for and adoration of your partner and, through him or her, the universe. Mutually circulate the accumulating sexual energies, sharing them and connecting with each other on every possible level. Build this ecstasy with repeated inner orgasm, drawing the inner energy up and giving it wholly back to your partner. This is the path to enlightenment through sex.

Karma and Sin

Karma and sin are the residual traces in consciousness of actions taken under the influence of lower desires. They are essentially similar concepts that are of great importance in sexual mysticism. Both, however, have been perverted into practical nonsense and desperately need to be rescued from the sloppy thinking inherent in our culture. There is nothing "evil" in either sin or karma. This perception is merely the result of dualistic tendencies that superimpose moral judgments on metaphysical concepts and cosmic principles. The word "sin" means error, not wickedness. It refers to an archer whose shot has missed its mark. When you stray from the path of your destiny, you sin. Karma is simply the result in your own life and consciousness of these actions.

You sin and create negative karma when your actions take you further away from your True Will. If you stay in abusive or emotionally unsatisfying relationships, fail to take action toward your real life goals, or allow your desires for comfort, safety, or momentary satisfaction to take you away from your appointed life path—this is the only sin you can ever really commit. And the results of these actions in your life are karma in its truest sense. There is no punishment for this from an authority above. The consequences in your mind and your life create the punishment. The solution is not to abandon the world in an act of renunciation, but rather to free yourself from your addiction to these lower desires. The remedy? Love.

The ancient libertine Gnostics who engaged in sexual activities felt it sinless, because they had freed themselves from the lower desires. It is desire, however, that launches magical energy and makes sexuality possible. If you have no desire for sex, it is unlikely that it will occur— unless you are pursued and acquiesce, in which case, you will most likely not enjoy the sex and it will create very little magical energy.

Desire does not disappear from the life of sexual magicians and mystics; it becomes a tool, a servant. Using desire to accomplish your True Will, or rather to embody that will, is an act of sacred magic. Accomplishment is meaningless in and of itself. Congruency of action, thought, and feeling is all that you can ever attain. Lust for some particular result, even if that result is your true destiny, is just as much enslavement to karma and sin as simply eating, drinking, and fucking yourself into oblivion.

Since your True Will always transcends your individual ego consciousness, the energy you direct toward your True Will is always mystical. And this is the key that transforms all of life into the Great Work. This is the alchemy of existence.

CHAPTER 10
Sexual Alchemy

Let him come through the first ordeal, & it will be to him as silver. Through the second, gold. Through the third, stones of precious water. Through the fourth, ultimate sparks of the intimate fire.

—*Liber AL vel Legis, III, 64-67*

Alchemy is a complicated and diffuse subject. There is no one authoritative text, philosophy, or process that defines it. Rather, it is a set of complex and multi-layered symbols that cannot be examined logically. These symbols lead in a non-rational way toward the transcendent, in an expanding kaleidoscope of metaphor and image. There are many types of physical and spiritual alchemy, with sexuality playing only a relatively minor role in most interpretations of the subject.

This chapter will not attempt to define alchemy, but rather will look at the evolutionary process of sexual awakening and empowerment through the lens of alchemical principles. We will briefly explore step-by-step methods for spiritual development through the seven basic processes of sexual alchemy. This is really just the practical application of all that we have explored in this book, a means of placing it within the context of a sort of ground plan for personal development within relationship.

There are many ways to approach the alchemical process. You can look at it as a simple a two-step process:

- Solve/divide
- Coagula/put back together

Or you can look at it as a three-step process that corresponds to the sacred name IAO:

- I/Isis (nature, prima materia)
- A/Apophis (destruction, putrefaction, or separation)
- O/Osiris (resurrection, conjunction, and perfection)

Or as a four step process that corresponds to colors:

- Albedo/whitening
- Nigredo/blackening
- Citrinitas/yellowing
- Rubedo/reddening

You can even see it as a twelve-step process that relates to the cycle of organic life:

- Calcination
- Solution
- Element separation
- Conjunction
- Putrefaction
- Coagulation
- Cibation
- Sublimation
- Fermentation
- Exaltation
- Augmentation
- Projection

However you look at it, the alchemical process comes down to transformation—changing something from its imperfect natural state to a more exalted state. By carefully taking this "something" apart and rebuilding it, you achieve its perfection. Although this is often described in popular literature as the physical process of changing lead into gold, there has also always been a spiritual component to the alchemical operation. By examining the work of our alchemical brethren in the East, we quickly discover that this spiritual process inherently involves sexual energy. Here, we will examine the seven-step process made famous in a very intriguing engraving from 1616 by S. Michelspacher (see figure 28). These seven steps are:

Calcination
Sublimation

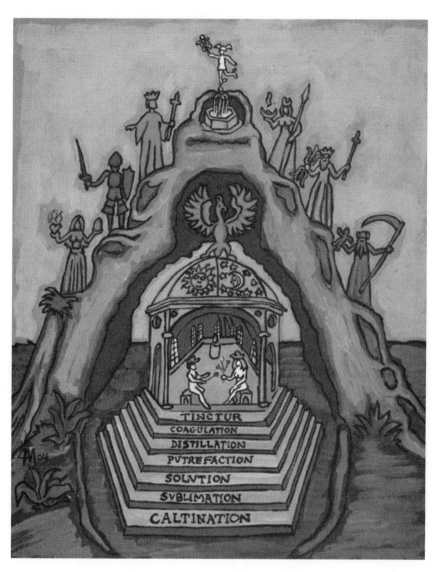

Figure 28. The seven alchemical steps

Solution
Putrefaction
Distillation
Coagulation
Tincture

For our purposes, sexual alchemy is really the alchemy of relationship, the process of interaction and growth discussed throughout this book. This interaction includes your relationships with others, but most important, it involves your relationship with the elements of your own being. Through the process of sexual alchemy, you discover your true self. There may be many layers of cultural garbage to sift through in order to discover your true self. We have all suffered damage, received bad advice, and absorbed negative conditioning throughout our lives. The alchemical process of self-discovery, however, can lead you progressively toward your real destiny.

STAGE 1

CALCINATION: *Heating to a high temperature, but without fusing, in order to drive off volatile matter or to effect changes. Reducing the prima materia to a fine ash.*

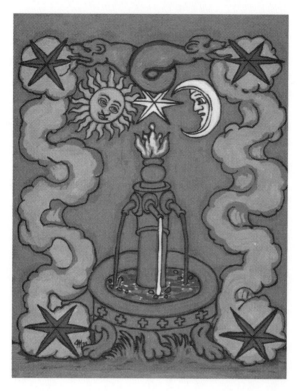

The first step in this inner alchemy of relationship is to look at yourself realistically, to examine who and what you are at the moment, and to begin "heating up" your consciousness by confronting your ego conflicts and self-doubts. Your goal is to destroy the status quo—the ego as it exists in its current state—through self-evaluation and introspection. This is a revolutionary step, but one you must undertake to evolve spiritually and sexually. You must recognize that you are not currently where you would like to be, or who you would like to be, and begin to take real steps toward transformation.

Related activities: The Magical Mirror of the Self (see page 13), Become Self-aware (see page 13), Know Your Sexual Self (see page 14), Building Your Personal Sexual History (see page 30), Defining Your Ideal Sexual Partner (see page 31)

STAGE 2

SUBLIMATION: *Passing material directly from the solid to the vapor state and condensing it back on a higher level. Diverting the expression of desire from its primitive form to one that is more effective.*

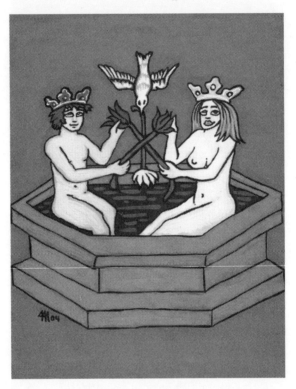

The second step is sublimation. This stage represents your first conscious redirecting of energy toward growth and transformation. Here you begin to discover your inner energies, your interior world, and your blockages. You can then begin to remove blocks, doubts, and fears, and direct your energies toward the higher level of being and sexual development that you desire. It is your quest directly into yourself, your soul's journey toward self-actualization.

Related activities: Entering a Magick Trance (see page 50), Breathing in Awareness and Energy (see page 52), Creating Inner Visualizations (see page 53), Accessing Your Body of Light (see page 54), Discovering Your True Will (see page 75), Magical Goals (see page 75), Magical Chastity (see pages 104, 122, 137, and 153)

STAGE 3

SOLUTION: *The process of homogeneously mixing the transforming materials into a single substance. The condition of being dissolved.*

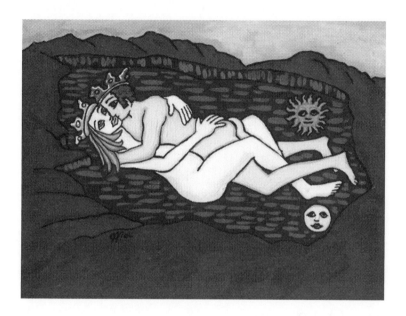

The next step is solution, sometimes called conjunction. In this process, you connect with your sexual partner and begin to connect to the polarities within yourself. You fuse together sexually, and fuse your inner and outer nature—the right and left hemispheres, the logical and imaginative faculties—into the alchemical "hermaphrodite" within. You begin to develop your interior powers, and a greater understanding of yourself.

Related activities: Relating to Your Animus and Anima (see page 84), Finding Your Sexual Energy Gateway (see page 90), Breathing in Your Sex Energy (see page 91), Invoking Your Holy Guardian Angel Autoerotically (see page 124), Invoking Your Holy Guardian Angel with a Partner (see page 139), Invoking Desired Qualities (see page 170), Invoking the Gods Autoerotically (see page 172), Invoking the Gods with Your Lover (see page 175)

STAGE 4

PUTREFACTION: *The blackening and decomposition of materials, a further separation of the impure from the pure.*

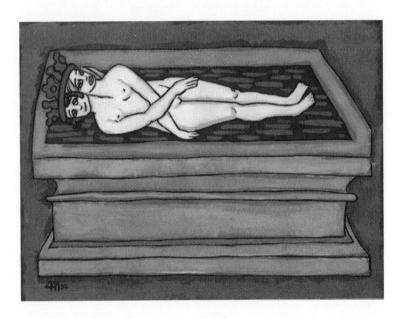

The next step is putrefaction, sometimes called fermentation. Here, you discover more inconsistencies and problems in your own nature through interaction with polarities. You allow these dark parts of yourself to emerge, and work through them. Your secret fears, doubts, and problems are unavoidable when you look at them through the lens of relationship. This stage also corresponds to the the Dark Night of the Soul. As you see yourself more clearly, the problems you secretly hold become more and more apparent. You must allow these parts of yourself to fall away.

Related activities: Discovering Your True Will (see page 75), Releasing Body Tension (see page 111), Breathing through Your Chakras (see page 112), Breathing in Chakra Energy (see page 113), Alternate-nostril Breathing (see page 114), Arousing Kundalini (see page 115), Invoking Sexual Archetypes (see page 201)

STAGE 5

DISTILLATION: *The process of purifying materials by*
successive evaporation and condensation

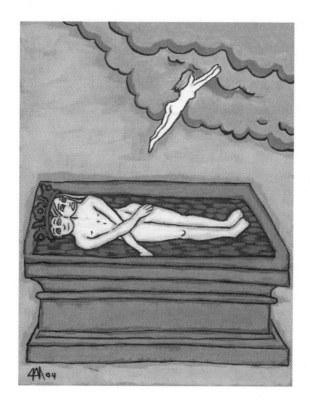

The next step in the process of sexual alchemy is distillation. Here, you
raise your energies actively toward the higher planes. You seek out experiences of transcendence and actively transform your internal energies
through invocation and increased self-awareness. It is also the transformation of your sexual energy into true spiritual power. It is the process
of freeing yourself of the negative elements that appeared in the phase
of putrefaction.

Related activities: The Lesser Heavenly Circle (see page 96), Breathing
through Your Chakras (see page 112), Alternate-Nostril Breathing (see
page 114), Arousing Kundalini (see page 115), Autoerotic Energetic
Practice (see page 122), Evoking Spirits (see page 207)

STAGE 6

COAGULATION: *the material gathers back together into a new coherent mass.*

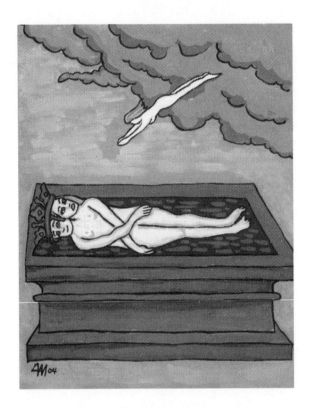

The next step is coagulation, in which the invoked forces and transformed energies come together within the body and the life of the alchemist.

Related activities: Mastering the Middle Pillar (see page 98), Creating Artificial Elementals (see page 210)

STAGE 7

TINCTURE: *the final solution of the medicinal substance, the extract of the process. The result.*

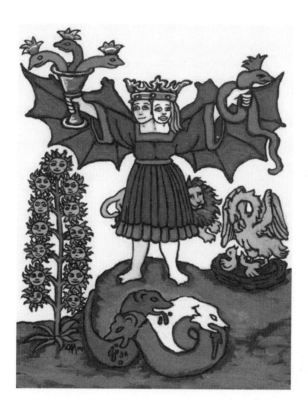

The last phase, tincture, is the final success of the work. It is the transformation of the self into an avatar of sexually enlightened divinity. It is the experience of cosmic consciousness, the transcendental illumination of sexual mysticism. It is also, of course, the fluids produced by the sex act, the elixir of life, the philosopher's stone.

Related activities: Thaumaturgy (see page 148)

You can also see this whole process playing out in simplified form within the thaumaturgic rite of sex magick itself:

- Calcination: You begin the sex act, concentrating on your goal, all other thoughts and experiences burned away by the ecstasy of sex.
- Sublimation: You begin to raise your inner energies. You draw energy within, and sublimate sexual energy to psychic energy, projecting it up to the heavens.
- Solution: You balance the ecstasy of the sex against the focus on your will, joining them together inseparably in the union with your lover.
- Putrefaction: You lose consciousness of your individuality as the repeating and ever-expansive ecstasies cause you to blackout.
- Distillation: You circulate and raise the sex energies further. The energies bubble up through you, continuing to transform animal passion into spiritual and magical force.
- Coagulation: The energy accumulates.
- Tincture: The elixir is released.

CHAPTER 11

Attracting Partners

Now think not to find them in the forest or on the mountain; but in beds of purple, caressed by magnificent beasts of women with large limbs, and fire and light in their eyes, and masses of flaming hair about them; there shall ye find them.

—*Liber AL vel Legis, II, 24*

The final secret of sex magick is a dark one that easily lends itself to both abuse and black magick. It is the art of seduction itself. This is the art of the lover, the ability to attract partners and seduce them into your bed. There is, of course, no way to define seduction clearly in words, because it is as much an art as painting, music, or poetry. The best we can do is provide a few basic magical and mundane principles for attracting lovers. These techniques range from simple magick spells, to the more direct tools of neuro-linguistic programming and practical psychological influence. As long as you remain honest, and don't attempt to deceive or take advantage of people, anything you do is acceptable.

Considering what a prolific lover Crowley was, and how many lovers, both male and female, he had throughout his life, he wrote very little about the art of seduction itself. Just a few stray sentences appear on this subject in his many thousands of pages of writings, and these few are, for the most part, sarcastic. In writing to one of his female students about the subject of "fascination," he said: "Dear me! Dear me! The world's indeed gone topsy turvy if you have to ask *me* for the secrets of Fascination!"[56] To men, he wrote: "We cannot exhaust the combinations of Lover's Chess, but we may enumerate the principal gambits: the Bouquet, the Chocolates, the Little Dinner, the Cheque-Book, the

Poem, the Motor by Moonlight, the Marriage Certificate, the Whip, and the Feigned Flight."[57] And elsewhere: "There is no need to knock the girl down, unless she refuses to do what you want, and she will always comply if you say a few nice things to her."[58] This is not particularly useful advice, even if it does contain an amusing little grain of truth.

You can start to attract mates magically by applying many of the techniques we have already discussed. Building up your own sexual abilities through energy work increases your confidence and desire for sex, and this magnetically attracts partners. Invoking positive qualities and divine beings empowers you, and you can easily create and evoke elementals and spirits to bring you lovers. Use all that we have discussed in these many pages, and you will quickly find yourself fulfilling your desires. All you need to do is go out and get into situations where you'll meet people.

If you are not regularly meeting potential mates already, you really must begin by expanding your social life. Join clubs. Go out after work with your work associates. Answer personal ads or place them. Make time and space in your life where it will be possible to meet lovers. This is really the most important thing you can do. If you are not meeting lovers, I guarantee it is mostly because you are not surrounding yourself with potential candidates. Get out of your house!

There are also many quite practical and simple ways of immediately becoming more attractive when you do start to meet people. The ability to hold a conversation with someone will carry you very far beyond the majority of humanity. Most people are nearly incapable of any kind of meaningful communication. And conversation is so incredibly easy. The secret to great conversation can be summed up in one word: Listen! Listen to what people are saying. Be interested in what they are talking about. Ask questions. Be interested in the answers. Talk about yourself, but don't always just bring topics back to yourself. Be genuinely interested. Don't be a liar. Be confident, but never arrogant or judgmental. Be funny, but not distracting or nervous.

You can establish rapport on many more subtle levels as well as through the art of conversation. By listening to your potential mates, you can discover all sorts of things about their desires. They will tell you about what they liked and did not like about past relationships, what their family dynamics were like growing up, how they interact with their friends, what they like and don't like about their friends' romantic relationships. You can integrate all of this information and match your behavior to your lover's desires. But you must be certain to match only those behaviors that you personally want in your own life, or you will just make yourself unhappy in the long run. When speaking with a potential mate, do not say that you like things that you do not like. This will only cause you misery. If you do not share common desires, move on.

One excellent way to establish rapport on a subtle, but extremely powerful, level is to observe and match a number of common tendencies in a potential mate's behavior.

These actions must be undertaken with a great deal of subtlety and care. Do not be obvious, or you will make your quarry nervous rather than comfortable. We all imitate each other's body language and behavior to a degree. It's just one of the many ways we communicate nonverbally. By being conscious of these habitual tendencies, you can have the power to create rapport with literally anyone.

Building Rapport

1. Assume a body posture or expression similar to the person with whom you want to establish a rapport. If your potential mate is sitting with legs crossed, mirror that. If his or her arms are folded, fold yours. If the person is upright or rigid, do this too. If he or she is slumped, try slumping. This will instantly put you in sympathy with your potential mate's attitude and emotional state.
2. Try imitating the breathing patterns of this person as well. Some people breathe high in the chest, others in the belly. Some breathe quickly, or shallowly, or deeply, or rhythmically. Match this, and you are well on your way to establishing rapport. Once you have established a subconscious connection through breathing, you can actually cause the person to shift that breathing pattern by shifting your own. This can have a powerful effect, without your potential mate even knowing about it, because your breathing strongly affects your mood and well-being.
3. Match the vocal tonality of the person to whom you are speaking. Is it high, sharp, loud, soft, low, or smooth? Try to speak in a similar or congruent tonality.
4. Observe the pace of your potential mate's speech. Is it slow or fast? Is it rhythmic or is it full of pauses? Try to match this as well.
5. How is his or her overall energy? Mellow? Tense? Enthusiastic? Be the same.
6. Are the person's movements graceful? Clunky? Clumsy? Jerky? Fast? Make yours that way too.

Magnetism

To attract lovers, you must increase your personal magnetism. There is really only one sexual game that people play—the game of cat and mouse. There are essentially two roles that can be played in any sexual and romantic courtship. You are either the pursuer or the pursued. It is terrible to say this, but, ideally, you want to be the pursued. This places you in the position of making all of the decisions for the relationship. I personally try to avoid this game altogether, laying my cards on the table and backing away if the other person is not interested in meeting me halfway. But, since it is hard to avoid this game, it is definitely best to be pursued. And the only way to be pursued is to create the perception that you are so great that your potential lover must make sure to be with you. To do this, you must have great charisma.

Charisma is really just a matter of being yourself, putting your best foot forward, and emphasizing your best qualities to others and in your own mind. There are things that are really great about you and these are the things you should emphasize in your self-talk and in your interactions with potential mates. Look your best when you are seeking a mate. Create a personal style that enhances your comfort and confidence. The following simple techniques are also extremely effective. It is unclear to me whether they are truly metaphysical in their action, or whether they just increase your own confidence from within. Either way, you may find them useful in creating more frequent and easy connections with potential lovers.

Projecting Animal Magnetism

1. Fix in your mind that you are going to be fascinating.
2. Visualize and feel this desire building within you, along with images of yourself being very charming and well-loved.
3. Build up this energy in yourself as a palpable glow of captivation that swirls around you.
4. Send this energy turning about around you, and imagine yourself glowing with a charismatic glamour.

Projecting Mental Influence

It is fairly easy to influence others by a simple projection of your will. This might seem to be very close to black magick, but as long as you are using it for positive reasons there is little harm.

1. Build up a field of magnetic and charismatic energy around you.
2. Project your thoughts silently out toward the target person on a wave of your magnetic energy: "You like me!" or "You want to know me!"
3. Imagine that your thoughts undulate like a wave of power into the person you wish to influence.

Standing Out in a Crowd

Standing out in a crowd is really a very simple matter and involves confidence, dress, posture, and positive energy.

1. Imagine and astrally build up a golden light, a blazing, shining Sun filling your aura, until you feel you are positively radiantly glowing. Become the Sun itself.
2. Allow yourself to feel big and bold and important. No one will be able to take his or her eyes off of you.
3. Don't stay in this state too long, as it will quickly turn you into an egomaniac.

Your Ideal Mate

If you are a wise sexual sorcerer, you won't want to attract just any lover; you will want to find that special lover who fulfills all your needs and whose needs you can entirely fulfill as well. You want to find your "soul mate." Of course, most of us are completely incapable of knowing what we really want until we have it in our hands, but you surely have some idea of the general qualities that make up your ideal mate.

Hopefully, you conducted the Defining Your Ideal Sexual Partner exercise (see page 31) and already have a list of these qualities at your disposal. I urge you to take another look at this list, and make adjustments and amendments to encompass your real needs and desires. Once you have this list in hand, you are well on your way to finding your ideal lover. The following steps can help you launch this desire out into the universe.

Finding Your Ideal Mate

1. Enter a magick trance.
2. Perform any opening ritual elements you like, then allow yourself to sit or lie down and move more deeply into the altered state.
3. In your mind, begin to make a detailed movie or series of images of your ideal mate and your interactions with this person. How will your lover treat you, talk to you, make love to you? Make this as exciting and dramatic as you possibly can—seeing the images, feeling the feelings, and hearing the sounds.
4. Play through these images until you have a coherent story of what you want to experience with your ideal lover.
5. Step into your movie and experience it in your body, as if you were really seeing, feeling, and hearing all of it with your ideal lover in the first person. Be *in* the experience.
6. Freeze the movie at the most exciting part, then step out of it and direct your attention to the globe of light above your head. See and feel yourself filling with this light. Feel love and power pass between you and your super-conscious, your Holy Guardian Angel.
7. Tell your Holy Guardian Angel that you want this desire to manifest, or something even better.
8. Arouse the kundalini sexual force within you, imagining that the movie containing your ideal mate is floating upward on a wave of energy into the light of your super-conscious. Know that your Holy Guardian Angel will handle the details of this manifestation. Travel up with the movie, experiencing an ecstatic Gnostic experience.
9. Return to normal consciousness.
10. Record your experience in your journal.

You can also add sexuality directly to this by masturbating throughout the process, and launching the movie into your super-conscious on a wave of orgasm. After you have conducted this exercise, be sure to take some real outward actions toward meeting this person. Make yourself available so your will can manifest. Keep your eyes open. Your soul mate is looking for you, too.

CONCLUSION

Magick and mysticism have as their backbone fundamental metaphysical structures that are inherent in us. They are the very nature of the universe as a whole. In fact, the truth of the mysteries of existence are often so internalized that many of us do not even recognize them. They may be so deeply imbedded in our subconscious or higher consciousness that we do not even have syllables to pronounce their undeniable truths.

These truths are available to us all, without books, through nothing but our own direct connection to them. Unfortunately, most of us are so enshrouded by the masks of consciousness—the highly charged emotional static that we each create to shield ourselves outwardly and inwardly—that we are unable to see them.

These truths are found in what C. G. Jung called the "collective unconscious." All cultures and theologies have addressed them in one way or another. Through the ages all mystical schools have agreed on some version of these fundamental principals:

0. The highest truth cannot be understood with words.
   The Tao that can be named is not the true Tao.
1. All things spring forth from an ultimate unity.
2. Out of unity comes polarity. Male and female of divine. The traditional symbol of Tao is the perfect hieroglyph.
3. A tri-form unity and polarity are both still considered unity. This can either be the offspring of a united pair, or a pair that together forms unity.
4. There is a spiritual place and/or condition that is totally separate from the rest of the universe.

5. All the power in the universe is at our disposal. Ask and ye shall receive, knock and it shall be opened unto you.
6. There are humans who are or become the incarnation of (or one with at least temporarily) the ultimate unity or god. Every human is capable of this unity (at least temporarily) and is at least able to perceive this unity.[59]
7. There are intelligent forces in the universe that are neither god, nor man, nor animal.
8. The universe functions according to rules, laws, and with mathematical precision.
9. There is a subtler realm, nonphysical, from which the universe manifests.
10. Waking life is like a dream and must be awoken from to experience true spiritual reality.

All the differences in the world's religions basically come down to disagreements about wording, names, and ceremonies associated with these principles. Since the first truth of all religion is that the highest truth cannot be understood by words, all differences are just plain nonsense.

NOTES

Introduction

1. Aleister Crowley, *Magick: Liber ABA* (York Beach, ME: Weiser Books, 1997), p. 165.
2. Jason Augustus Newcomb, *The New Hermetics* (York Beach, ME: Weiser Books, 2004), p. 2.
3. The sexual sorcerer knows that manipulation and obsession ultimately enslave both partners, and so prefers the path of freedom and ecstasy above all.
4. H. P. Blavatsky, *The Secret Doctrine* Vol. 1 (Pasadena, CA: Theosophical University Press, 1988), p. 192.
5. Blavatsky, *The Secret Doctrine* Vol. 2, p. 211.
6. Crowley, *Magick: Liber ABA*, p. 276
7. Crowley, *Magick: Liber ABA*, p. 661.
8. Crowley, *Magick: Liber ABA*, p. 493.
9. There are most likely people who will find this whole concept offensive, since I am quoting "Holy Books," Crowley's divinely inspired writings. How could they contain such obvious errors? But it must be remembered that the divine inspires us within our own cultural context. Hindus receive Hindu-related inspirations, Jews receive Jewish inspirations, and Christians receive Christian inspirations. It is the same divine that informs all these visions, but they are filtered and colored by the cultural milieu in which they are received. Crowley's subconscious had it in mind that left-hand-path adepts were evil, so his divine consciousness spoke to him in those terms.
10. C. W. Leadbeater, Edward Maitland, Anna Kingsford, Krishnamurti, Annie Besant, etc.
11. These terms describe a metaphysical energy present in the reproductive

fluids, which is essentially equivalent to the life force or magick force. There are so many words for this mystical substance that it can get quite dizzying. In essence, they are all one phenomena.

CHAPTER 1

12. This potential is probably reserved for those adepts who have truly balanced the foundations of the inner temple and can really see in every idea its opposite as an essential part if itself. This accomplished, all things are sacred, from the highest samadhi to the deepest depths of depravity and excrement.
13. Ireneaus, *Against all Heresies*, *www.gnostic.org*.
14. Farrar, Janet and Stewart, *A Witches Bible* (London: Phoenix, 1984), Part 2, p. 37.
15. Aleister Crowley, *Magick: Liber ABA* (York Beach, ME: Weiser Books, 1997), p. 588.

CHAPTER 2

16. Randolph, *Sexual Magic.*
17. It is interesting to note that both the twentieth-century German mage Franz Bardon and Randolph use the terms "volt" and "fluid condensers," and they are just about the only writers who do. They use them for slightly different meanings, but it shows that the reach of Randolph's system extended into far places. In Randolph's case, a "volt" means a willed force for accomplishing a desire that is placed into an object—like a small figure stored in an insulated jar.
18. The interested reader can explore these in Joscelyn Godwin, Christian Chanel, and John P. Deveney, *The Hermetic Brotherhood of Luxor* (York Beach, ME: Weiser Books, 1995).
19. Crowley, *Magick: Liber ABA*, p. 208.
20. Crowley, *Magick: Liber ABA*, p. 663. A "fiat" is a decree, in other words the expression of your magical will through the orgasm. The "day of Be-with-Us" may imply that you have raised your consciousness to the realm of the gods. Fiat is also a Latin acronym for the combination of the four elements: flotus, igni, aquae, terrae (air, fire, water, earth).
21. Crowley, *Magick: Liber ABA*, p. 267.
22. Crowley, *Magick: Liber ABA*, p. 267.
23. In this regard, the two operators are Nuit and Hadit, and the sexual fluids are Ra Hoor Khuit.
24. Crowley, *Magick: Liber ABA*, footnote, p. 157.
25. Aleister Crowley, *Liber Aleph* (York Beach, ME: Weiser Books, 1991), p. 82.
26. Crowley, *Magick: Liber ABA*, pp. 567–568.
27. See particularly "De Formula Tota," in Crowley, *Liber Aleph*, p. 86.
28. Crowley very often conducted his sex magick with non-magical

women, most often prostitutes. It is questionable whether they were at all aware of what he was doing. So, we can take it from this that Crowley felt that, as long as he was concentrating, it didn't matter what the prostitute was thinking.

29. Scott Michaelson (ed.), *Portable Darkness* (New York: Harmony Books, 1989), pp. 166–167.

30. You can also read my first book, *21st Century Mage*, which focuses entirely on the subject.

Chapter 3

31. Randolph, *Sexual Magic*, p. 48

32. Aleister Crowley, *Magick: Liber ABA* (York Beach, ME: Weiser Books, 1998), pp. 206–207.

33. H. P. Blavatsky, *Theosophical Glossary*, Sleep of Siloam entry.

34. Aleister Crowley, *Portable Darkness* (New York: Harmony Books, 1989), p. 165.

35. Aleister Crowley, *Liber Aleph* (York Beach, ME: Weiser Books, 1991), p. 18.

36. Crowley, *Magick: Liber ABA*, p. 523.

37. Jason Newcomb, *The New Hermetics* (York Beach, ME: Weiser Books, 2004), pp. 83–88. For more information on the subject, please visit *www.newhermetics.com*.

38. In yogic philosophy, this is expressed as the concepts of *Isvara* and *Atman*. Though the same existence, Isvara is god as we look at him in worship. Atman is god as we realize him in our own transcendence. Until we have realized our identity with god, god has all these perfect infinite qualities. Once we have transcended thought and obtained divine identity, there are no qualities.

39. Crowley, *Magick: Liber ABA*, p. 137.

40. Raphael Patai, *Hebrew Goddess* (Detroit: Wayne State University Press, 1990).

41. See Crowley, *Magick: Liber ABA*, p. 63 (footnote), pp. 137–141, and p. 153.

42. It is also interesting that they are quite similar to Paschal Beverly Randolph's Volantia, Decretism, and Tirauclairism, at least in practice. These are all also quite similar to the concepts of *kriya* (action), *iccha* (will), and *gnana* (knowledge) in yoga philosophy.

Chapter 4

43. Wilhelm Reich, *Character Analysis* (New York, Pocket Books, 1976), p. 434.

44. See Aleister Crowley, *Magick: Liber ABA* (York Beach, ME: Weiser Books, 1998), p. 569, or *The Book of Lies* (York Beach, ME: Weiser Books, 1986), p. 60.

45. You may wish to consult my *21st Century Mage*, S. L. Mathers's *The Book of the Sacred Magic of Abramelin the Mage*, or Aleister Crowley's *Liber VIII* in regard to this work.

CHAPTER 5

46. Aleister Crowley, *Liber Aleph* (York Beach, ME: Weiser Books, 1991), p. 24.
47. Crowley, *Liber Aleph*, p. 144.
48. For two different versions of this rite, see Crowley's *Magick: Liber ABA, Book 4*, pp. 513–522 and Stephen Flowers's *Hermetic Magic*, (York Beach, ME: Weiser Books, 1995), pp. 182–183.
49. Crowley, *Magick: Liber ABA*, p. 570, or *The Book of Lies*, pp. 82–83.

CHAPTER 6

50. See note 20 in chapter 2.
51. Aleister Crowley, *The Magical Record of the Beast 666* (London: Duckworth, 1972), pp. 3–82.
52. See Crowley, *Magick: Liber ABA*, pp. 195–200 for a discussion of these elements of ritual.
53. By the way, my girlfriend called!
54. A remarkably similar technique of creating monogram sigils can also be found in Agrippa's *Three Books of Occult Philosophy* (London: Gregory Moule, 1651), p. 444.

CHAPTER 9

55. Aleister Crowley, *Liber Aleph* (York Beach, ME: Weiser Books, 1992), p. 28.

CHAPTER 11

56. Aleister Crowley, *Magick Without Tears* (Phoenix, AZ: New Falcon Publications, 1991), p. 184.
57. Aleister Crowley, *Magick: Liber ABA* (York Beach, ME: Weiser Books, 1998), p. 221.
58. Crowley, *Magick: Liber ABA,* ch. 11, p. 202.

CONCLUSION

59. As in those theologies wherein man is but a creation of the ultimate god, and unable to ascend to that state himself.

BIBLIOGRAPHY AND SUGGESTED READINGS

Anand, Margo. *The Art of Sexual Ecstasy*. New York: G. P. Putnam's Sons, 1989.

Bardon, Franz. *Initiation into Hermetics*. Wuppertal, Germany: Ruggeberg-Verlag, 1993.

Carroll, Peter. *Liber Kaos*. York Beach, ME: Samuel Weiser Books, 1992.

———. *Liber Null and Psychonaut*. York Beach, ME: Samuel Weiser Books, 1987.

Chia, Mantak. *Healing Love through the Tao*. Huntington, NY: Healing Tao Books, 1986.

———. *Taoist Secrets of Love*. Santa Fe, NM: Aurora Press, 1984.

Crowley, Aleister. *777 and Other Qabalistic Writings*. York Beach, ME: Weiser Books, 1973.

———. *The Book of Lies*. York Beach, ME: Weiser Books, 1991.

———. *The Book of Thoth*. York Beach, ME: Weiser Books, 1974.

———. *Commentaries on the Holy Books*. York Beach, ME: Weiser Books, 1996.

———. *The Equinox* Vols. 1–10. York Beach, ME: Weiser Books, 1999.

———. *Liber Aleph*. York Beach, ME: Weiser Books, 1991.

———. *Magical Diaries of Aleister Crowley*. York Beach, ME: Weiser Books, 1996.

———. *The Magical Record of the Beast 666*. London: Duckworth, 1972.

———. *Magick: Liber ABA*. York Beach, ME: Weiser Books, 1997.

———. *Magick Without Tears*. Phoenix, AZ: New Falcon Publications, 1991.

———. *The Scented Garden of Abdullah*. Chicago: The Teitan Press, 1991.

———. *The Vision and the Voice*. York Beach, ME: Weiser Books, 1998.

Culling, Louis. *Sex Magick*. St. Paul, MN: Llewellyn Books, 1989.

Duquette, Lon Milo. *The Magick of Thelema*. York Beach, ME: Weiser Books, 1993.

———. *Enochian Sex Magick*. Phoenix, AZ: New Falcon Publications, 1991.

————. *Understanding Aleister Crowley's Thoth Tarot*. Boston: Weiser Books, 2003.

Farrar, Janet and Stewart. *A Witches Bible*. London: Phoenix, 1984.

Flowers, Stephen. *Hermetic Magic*. York Beach, ME: Weiser Books, 1995.

Gawain, Shakti. *Creative Visualization*. New York: Bantam Books, 1978.

Godwin, Joscelyn, Christian Chanel, and John P. Deveney. *The Hermetic Brotherhood of Luxor*. York Beach, ME: Weiser Books, 1995.

Gray, Henry. *Anatomy, Descriptive and Surgical*. Philadelphia: Running Press, 1974.

Hine, Phil. *Condensed Chaos*. Tempe, AZ: New Falcon Publications, 1995.

Jou, Tsung Hwa. *The Tao of Meditation*. Warwick, NY: Tai Chi Foundation, 1983.

Jung, Carl G. *Alchemical Studies*. Princeton, NJ: Princeton University Press, 1967.

————. *The Archetypes and the Collective Unconscious*. Princeton, NJ: Princeton University Press, 1969.

King, Francis. *Sexuality, Magic, and Perversion*. Los Angeles: Feral House, 2002.

Knight, Richard and Thomas Wright. *A History of Phallic Worship*. New York: Dorset Press, 1992.

Lidell, Lucy. *The Sivananda Companion to Yoga*. New York: Fireside, 1983.

Mead, G.R.S. *Thrice Great Hermes: Studies in Hellenistic Theosophy and Gnosis, Volume II*. London: Theosophical Publishing Society, 1906.

Michaelson, Scott, ed. *Portable Darkness*. New York: Harmony Books, 1989.

Newcomb, Jason Augustus. *21st Century Mage*. Boston, MA: Weiser Books, 2002.

————. *The New Hermetics*. Boston, MA: Weiser Books, 2004.

Randolph, Pascal Beverly. *Sexual Magic*. New York, Magickal Childe Publishing, 1988.

Regardie, Israel. *The Complete Golden Dawn System of Magic*. Phoenix, AZ: New Falcon Publications, 1990.

————. *The Golden Dawn*. St. Paul, MN: Llewellyn Books, 1989.

————. *The Middle Pillar*. St. Paul, MN: Llewellyn Books, 1987.

Reich, Wilhelm. *Character Analysis*. New York: Pocket Books, 1976.

————. *The Function of the Orgasm*. New York: Farrar, Strauss and Giroux, 1973.

Roob, Alexander. *Alchemy and Mysticism*. New York: Taschen, 2001.

Steinbrecher, Edwin. *The Inner Guide Meditation*. York Beach, ME: Weiser Books, 1988.

Wang, Robert, *Qabalistic Tarot*, (York Beach, ME: Weiser Books, 1987)

Wilson, Robert Anton. *Prometheus Rising*. Phoenix, AZ: Falcon Press, 1983.

ABOUT THE AUTHOR

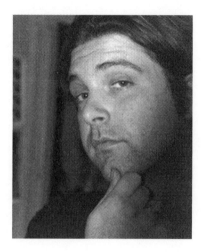

Jason Augustus Newcomb is a writer and artist who has worked with
the powers of the mind and consciousness-altering practices for many
years. He lives in Florida, but travels across the U.S. giving lectures and
workshops. He is the author of *21st Century Mage* and *The New Hermetics*.

TO OUR READERS

Weiser Books, an imprint of Red Wheel/Weiser, publishes books across the entire spectrum of occult and esoteric subjects. Our mission is to publish quality books that will make a difference in people's lives without advocating any one particular path or field of study. We value the integrity, originality, and depth of knowledge of our authors.

Our readers are our most important resource, and we appreciate your input, suggestions, and ideas about what you would like to see published. Please feel free to contact us, to request our latest book catalog, or to be added to our mailing list.

Red Wheel/Weiser, LLC
P.O. Box 612
York Beach, ME 03910-0612
www.redwheelweiser.com